IN SEARCH OF HELEN
FROM TWO LOCKS

by Jack McBride White
with Sidney Starliper

ASHLEIGH-REID, PUBLISHERS

In Search of Helen from Two Locks
Ashleigh-Reid, Publishers
First Edition, October 2020

ISBN: 9798677238239

Cover Design: Andrea White
Cover Photos: Helen Starliper and Dam 5 on the C&O Canal
(All photos provided by courtesy of the Starliper family,
except where otherwise noted.)

Cover photo of Dam 5 by Stephen Walker: unsplash.com/@stphnwlkr

DEDICATION

To my mother, Helen Starliper, found at last.

~ Sid Starliper

For Sid and Mike, and for all the Springfield nurses,
who worked so hard for so long taking care of
troubled souls like Helen Starliper.

~ Jack White

Special tribute to Charles "Sonny" Starliper,
who paved the way through his research and writings
and would be so happy to see the results.
You are missed, Brother.

The truth is the truth — no matter.

SALLY BOSWELL (DAUGHTER OF HELEN'S BROTHER
HARRY RANDOLPH SMALL)

CONTENTS

IN SEARCH OF HELEN FROM TWO LOCKS

Sometimes deep in the nucleus of cells, a malformed monster lurks, a biological mutant that can sit dormant for years before rising from its slumber. When and if it does, the monster can wreak havoc.

JOHN PERRITANO, *NATIONAL GEOGRAPHIC*, 2019

THE COLONY

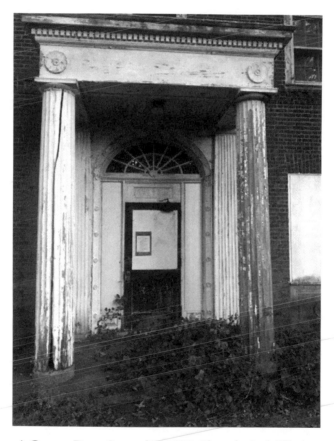

A Cottage Door, September 2020. Photo by Jack White.

COTTAGE 5

October, 1952

Let's go straight to Helen and that Wednesday night when the fever hit. Her name was Helen Starliper then, but she was born Helen Elizabeth Small in 1913 and grew up in a beautiful place near a dam right on the C&O Canal in Washington County, Maryland. They called the area Two Locks, and during the first 20 years of her life, Helen's back yard ended at a rock cliff, thirty or forty feet high, that faced out over the Potomac River toward West Virginia.

But now it was October 1, 1952, sometime before midnight, and Helen hadn't been home in a long time. For almost a year, she had lain in bed, surrounded by other beds filled with other women, all much older than she was.

She was in Cottage 5, in a place they called the colony, when the fever hit. It came on suddenly, and soon she stared out at nothing through wet, glassy eyes. She was hot to the touch and breathing hard. On Thursday morning, her temperature crossed 105 and stayed there, right at the edge of human endurance. Her heart raced 140 times a minute, while nurses worked frantically to bring the fever down.

They put an ice cap on her head. They bathed her with sponges and tepid water and fed her crushed ice. She hadn't moved much in the past year or so, and her bones had pushed up through her skin, causing bed sores, or what the nurses called "pressure points." They were open and ugly and painful and spread across her back and down to her buttocks.

They cleaned them with water, peroxide, and something called Balsam Peru. They covered the sores with sterile dressings and bathed them with light from special infrared lamps, two minutes at a time. They fed her small amounts of milk and water and food. She had trouble swallowing and sometimes threw everything back up.

They fed her an antibiotic called Gantrisin, something else for nausea, and Demerol for pain.

She was 39. She had seven children. In July of 1950, when she first arrived at the huge facility where she lay now, she was a different person. She smiled. She ate well. She could walk, at least a bit, in her odd way. She could listen and respond and maybe get out a word or two.

You might say she was older then. She was 36. But for several years, she'd been slipping backward through the phases of human development, and now, like a newborn, she was helpless.

The colony was actually called the Epileptic Colony, although Helen did not have epilepsy. They also called it Clark Circle in honor of Dr. Clement Clark, the hospital superintendent, who had it built for insane epileptics in the 1920s.

By the time Helen arrived, there were fewer epileptics to care for, but many more patients of every other type, and so they put the colony to other uses.

The colony's still there on the grounds of the Springfield Hospital Center in Maryland, just outside the town of Sykesville. There are seven buildings in the colony forming a small circle around a plot of grass.

A respected Baltimore architect named Henry Powell Hopkins designed them. He got to work in 1924 and finished with Cottage 5 in 1938.

A lot has changed since then. The hospital is much smaller. The men's wards up a distant hill from the colony are abandoned, overgrown, and crumbling. The women's wards are mostly abandoned, and the buildings in the colony are all empty. They form a little ghost village, where weeds push up through cracked macadam and gnarled trees grow tall in the circle of grass. There are old fire hydrants painted white. There's gravel and big white rocks and broken branches on the grass and the paths.

The cottages are mostly brick. There are two floors. Vines climb up the walls and droop down from rooftops. All the first-floor windows are covered with wood that's painted white. The doors are locked. Hammered onto each door is a piece of unpainted plywood. Hammered onto the plywood is a hard-plastic sleeve of sorts, and inside the sleeve is a white sheet with words and boxes. Some boxes are checked, which means there's asbestos inside.

A brick path leads up to the door of each cottage. The bricks are broken and partly covered with weeds. There are white columns on each side of each entryway, except for Cottage 5. Most of the paint has chipped off the columns. The architecture is something called Georgian Revival.

When the fever hit, Helen had been in Cottage 5 nearly a year, mostly in bed, watched over by nurses who worked 12-hour shifts for little pay.

The nurses dreaded losing a patient and knew they were in danger of losing Helen. Her pulse was erratic. She gasped for air. She arched her neck and grimaced whenever anyone moved her arms or head.

At midnight on October 4, with her temperature at 104 and her heart beating 96 times a minute, Helen smiled at the nurse taking care of her. The nurse wrote it down.

"Smiled. Resting."

And then at 8 a.m., with the fever down to 103, her color better, and her heartbeat at 104, the nurse wrote the following in the upper right margin of the paper where she reported Helen's progress.

"Patient was able to talk."

That's all. Five words scribbled 70 years ago, but so frustrating, so intriguing, and maybe something like a small miracle.

3

THE BEGINNING

I found my mother.

Helen has her arm around me. We walk together.
We cry together. We laugh together. We smile together.

Please tell the world.

SID STARLIPER, JANUARY 18, 2020

It's September 2020, nearing the end of a dry, sizzling summer after a long, wet, lousy spring. A lot has changed since I started this book in 2018. We're in the midst of a global pandemic that shows little sign of abating, at least in the United States, where more than 200,000 people have died. Every day the number goes up.

The governor closed Maryland, where I live, for all but essential business, and we spent several weeks on lockdown. The roads emptied. The bars and restaurants locked their doors. Everyone in Walmart, and anyplace else that stayed open, so-called essential businesses, wore masks to keep from spreading the disease. We're coming out of it now. Maybe. People are tired of wearing masks. Fighting about them. But the virus doesn't care. The virus has no mind, no heart, no soul, no sense of its own existence. It just knows how to make copies of itself.

The virus causes a disease called COVID-19. The official name of the virus is SARS-CoV-2. Mostly we call it the coronavirus, or the novel coronavirus. It's a strange snippet of something called RNA that

4

may have started life (if you could call it that) in a so-called wet market in Wuhan, China, where it crossed over from animal to person and quickly ran rampant, bringing death and misery and a sudden economic recession.

Only scientists can see the virus and only with years of knowledge and training, great skill, and powerful tools.

It's nearly unbelievable, when you think about it. It's also indisputably true, that tiny invisible things, mindless and unaware, can grow and mutate and kill us in great numbers. Near the end of World War I, in 1918, a new strain of flu killed more soldiers in much less time than all the millions of bullets and shells and canisters of gas the various armies threw at one another combined.

Which brings me to Helen and her daughter Patsy and to Sid and all his brothers and sisters and how something even smaller than our coronavirus shaped their lives and led to the story I'm about to tell you.

But this isn't a book about biology or science, the cruelty of invisible things, or our struggles to understand and defeat them. It's about a man in his seventies trying to piece together the story of his mother's life and death, 70 years after it happened, with nothing but scattered fragments of information to work with.

His name is Sid Starliper. Helen is his mother. He can't remember her, and if not for a school bus at an intersection outside a Bob Evans in Frederick, Maryland, he would still know almost nothing about her. But there was a bus, and ever since he saw that bus, Sid has been searching without pause for Helen.

THE BUS

Did I get on the school bus?
Am I riding on the bus and don't know it?

SID STARLIPER, JANUARY 18, 2020

First thing Sid does each day is say, "Good morning, Mom, I love you." Each night before bed, he says, "Good night, Mom, I love you." No, she's not there. At least not in any visible form.

Sid was born in 1943. Helen rode out of his life in the backseat of a sheriff's car in 1950. His full name is Sidney Allen Starliper. He grew up in Clear Spring, Maryland, and lives in Frederick, Maryland now. He has mostly white hair, combed straight back and thinning. He wears hearing aids and often a baseball cap. He's a nice guy, kindhearted, considerate, and sensitive, and one day he walked into Bob Evans in Frederick and his life took a sudden, unexpected turn.

He was in the early days of retirement after 40 years of building houses. He didn't have any big plans. He was more worried about how to work out the money than anything else.

Then he was in that diner. Old songs came out of old speakers in the ceiling. Dishes clanked. Waitresses scrawled on little pads. He ate sausage gravy and pancakes by a window that faced a crowded street. He noticed a very old lady sitting nearby. She was smiling and laughing with a younger couple. The younger couple were about Sid's age. Sid assumed the old lady was the man's mother.

And that's when he looked up through the window and saw a school bus stuck in traffic right in front of him. Just a standard yellow bus with big letters on the side and windows full of kids. Maybe it had something to do with the old woman, he's not sure, but when he saw the bus, he had a sudden thought.

"How did my mother get to school?"

For some reason, he felt compelled to ask the lady that same question. He walked over to her table, pardoned himself for interrupting, and asked, "When you were a kid, how did you get to school?"

He never got her name. He did get her age. 98. When Sid's mother was 10, this woman was five. She grew up in California. Sometimes she walked to school and sometimes she rode the horse. When she rode the horse, it dropped her off and found its way back home. Sid hugged her and paid for the family's breakfast.

By the time he left Bob Evans, he couldn't think of anything except Helen. Who was she? What happened to her? Why couldn't he remember her? All he had was one unpleasant memory, hazy, sort of a bad dream, maybe recurring, that he couldn't quite bring all the way back. In the memory, Helen's crying in the dark. She says one word.

"Whitey." She repeats it while she cries.

Whitey was Sid's father, Charles Starliper. And the reason Sid could hear Helen is because Sid was in the room with his parents, lying in an undersized bed he shared with his brothers Bob and Dave, so close that, if he wanted, he could reach out and touch Helen's hand. And he thinks he knows why Helen cried.

"My dad was a butcher in a grocery store. In the back, they would bring in the sides of beef, or whatever, and he would process that, cut it up, make hamburger, and every night after work he'd go out drinking. We were asleep when he'd come home, and he would wake her up, and then I would hear the crying."

A GOOD PLACE TO DIE

I want to live forever, but if I have to die,
this would be a good place to do it.

SID STARLIPER

Two Locks, Easter 2016

Helen went into the asylum in July 1950, and Sid never heard her voice again. He knew that he was seven when she left and nine when she died. He didn't know much about why she went, or what happened to her while she was there, or why no one ever took him to visit her. He knew that the place where she died was still there, but he had never wanted to see it.

He didn't remember the day she left. He didn't remember if she kissed him goodbye. He didn't remember their last conversation. He didn't remember any conversation.

She died and Sid went on over six decades, working and raising daughters, until he went to Bob Evans that day. And then nothing much mattered except his search through the past for traces of Helen, wondering all the while how he could forget her so completely. He didn't know anything.

He didn't know about her early years on the C&O Canal. He didn't know about her mom and dad and brothers and sisters. He didn't know how she met Whitey, or what her marriage was like. He didn't know why they took her away.

It was shocking. He had a mother for seven years. He must have loved her. But then she left. His life, his memory. And now, suddenly, all these years later, he couldn't stop thinking about her. He felt an overwhelming sense of love and guilt and responsibility.

He quickly enlisted his family in his search. He has three daughters. Holly is the second. He visited her that night. Holly's daughter, Hannah, started up Google Earth on her computer, and they all sat around till midnight trying to find the old house along the canal where Helen grew up. But the house was small and smothered in weeds and brush and trees, and Google's satellites couldn't see it.

It didn't matter. Sid knew where it was. It had been sitting empty and ignored by the side of the road since 1979, and in March of 2016, on Easter Sunday, he went back to Helen's old house.

There were better days he could have done this. His sister Beverly was expecting him at noon for an Easter meal with the family. But Sid couldn't wait. He went to church. And then, without much time to spare, he hurried over to the river and the house where Helen grew up.

It was nice once. He'd seen pictures. It was solid and perfectly maintained, with a picket fence all around and a neatly cultivated garden. At one time, ten or eleven of them had lived there, but by 1950, everyone had moved out except Helen's oldest brother, a reclusive veteran of the First World War, who didn't talk much and resembled a man in his fifties when he was only 35.

His name was Bob Small. He never married, and Sid had no memory of him, and not the slightest inkling that when Bob was 24, the Army sent him to France and straight into the bloodiest battle in American history. Bob was with the 313th Infantry Regiment of the Army's 79th Division. They called themselves Baltimore's Own. They called the battle the Meuse-Argonne Offensive.

9

It began before dawn on September 26, 1918, and lasted 47 days. More than 25,000 Americans died. Bob had no experience and was thrown immediately into the thick of it. He lasted nine days before he was carried from the battlefield to a hospital in France.

When Bob died in 1979 it had been sixty years since May of 1919, when he came home through Newport News, Virginia, on the packed troop ship Antigone, with thousands of other soldiers. The federal government bought the canal and all the land around it in 1938 and turned it into a national park in 1971. Shortly after Bob's death, they took the house and gave the family $18,000 to split up.

By that Easter when Sid showed up at the old house, it had been empty 35 years. Helen's parents had owned it since 1903 and had lived in it several years before that with Helen's great aunt. It had once been sturdy and filled with nice things. The furniture was big and heavy and antique and may have dated back to the 18th century. The flatware was pewter. The tables were topped with marble. The condiment set was silver. The bottles that held vinegar and oil were crystal.

Outside was a small barn filled with tools all neatly arranged. There were chicken boxes surrounded by a fence. There was a wash-house, where Helen's dad would hang and salt half a beef each winter to provide meat for the cold months.

Sid has a cousin named Shirley Talhelm, who was born in 1934 and lives in Canada now. She grew up nearby, visited often, and re-members the old house and just about everything else in amazing detail.

"I can remember going up the garden path and through the gate, and they had a brick on the gate and a chain, and the brick would pull the gate closed, and I can still, to this day, hear that gate when it closed.

"And there was always a bucket of lime water out there to white-wash the fence. There was always a brush there, so they'd go by, when the women had time, or sometimes they sent we kids out there, and they'd just whitewash a couple pickets at a time.

"All up along the fence were raspberry bushes. When you went up the garden path there was a grape arbor with seats, and the women used to sit in there, and they'd go out and pick peas and beans or whatever, and they'd sit in there and snap the beans or hull the peas.

"There was a shrub by the walkway going into the front of the house. I can still smell that thing. It must be a hundred years old. It was there as long as I can remember. And you'd go out the back gate and down over the hill, and there was the river. We played down on those rock cliffs, and we swam in the river."

But except for the rocks and the river, that was all gone when Sid showed up that Sunday, all the bureaus and tables, all the crystal and silver and pewter and nice furniture passed down through generations, all the chickens and berries and fences and flowers. Everything except the collapsing structure, wood and nails and stone mixed with blown branches and dead leaves, all of it gray or brown.

And now came Sid, like some soldier back from a long war only to find his home in rubble and all his family gone.

The house leaned just a few feet off the road. There was no traffic. There were no sidewalks. The road was barely wide enough for cars heading in opposite directions to squeeze by each other. There were birds and squirrels and the river, just beyond the trees that were filling in after another dead winter.

There were no doors in the house. There were window frames, but no glass. The front stood. There was a doorway. There were still four walls.

Sid worked his way through the thick weeds and thorny brambles between his maroon Honda and the house. His heart beat fast. He looked inside. He had been here before once or twice, but that was long ago before he really cared.

11

Now it all hit him. All these years, his mother's house stood here, slowly falling apart, not meaning a thing to him. She spent years in there, hundreds of weeks, thousands of days, most of her life.

She was there when her terrified brother climbed up a ladder 3,000 miles away, and stumbled out into a whirlwind of shrapnel, bullets, smoke, and gas. She was there through the great flu of 1918 and 1919 that started near the end of the war and added more millions to the millions already dead. She was there through the Roaring Twenties and the Great Depression, and right up to the brink of the second great war.

She did homework in there. She had friends over. She heard the whistle of distant trains and the blast of tin horns and bugles as boat captains announced their pending arrival at the various locks along the canal. She sang Christmas carols in there, while an older sister played piano.

Now, beyond the missing front door, there was no first floor, just a drop, ten feet or so, down to the cellar. There was old wood down there and nature and all the things that dropped as the roof fell in. Enough light made its way down that he could see the black foundation stones.

It was all very solid once. Men who might have fought in the war between the states and carried bayonets into battle, or come over from Ireland to build the canal, spent hard days carrying rocks up from the river and fixing them in place and building the foundation of a life where Helen's family would grow and thrive for several decades, before slowly shrinking down to nothing, as one strange tragedy followed another.

Sid fought his way up to the entrance. Just a few feet in was a stairway. He wanted to take it upstairs, where there were still floors.

"But to do that," he says, "I had to jump from the front door entrance across a three-foot landing that wasn't there anymore."

Three feet isn't that long, but there was another problem. The stairs were right there, just across that small chasm and the long drop to the cellar, but the stairs were only attached to the wall on the right side. There was a wall on the left, but the stairway wasn't attached to it anymore. It hung there.

There was a good chance that when Sid propelled himself across the drop and hit the steps, the old stairway would collapse and he would end up in the cellar. There was a chance the stairs, the wall they'd been attached to, or maybe even the whole house would fall down on top of him. All anyone would find was his car and a pile of rubble, and wonder, "What ever happened to Sid Starliper?"

There was also the fact that Sid was 74. He used to be center half on his high school soccer team, a starting pitcher on the baseball team, a forward on the basketball team, but that was long ago. He could still move well enough, but he was hardly nimble and couldn't remember the last time he jumped over anything where if he didn't make it, there was a decent chance he would die. It just didn't seem all that smart to make that short jump.

But he did. And landed fine. The staircase held. And now he had another somewhat terrible idea.

"Insane as it was to climb a set of stairs that were just hanging there with no support, my adrenalin took over, and I never considered the danger."

There were about ten steps, just plain wooden planks. His mom must have climbed them thousands of times. When she left home it was 1937, and she was 24. Now her son, who was 50 years older than that, stood at the bottom and looked up. The stairway was steep. There was no good reason to expect the steps to hold. But Sid went right up and didn't stop till he reached the second floor and looked up where the roof used to be.

The floor was bare wood. There were gaps between boards. Some were missing, and there was still a good chance he could end up in the cellar with most of the house on top of him. He stepped carefully into each room. Once, they'd been clean and filled with big, old, heavy furniture.

Sid's heart beat fast. He was a bit out of breath, and he was happy.

"It was very emotional. Here I am, up there on the second floor looking up into the sky, and I'm standing almost in all three bedrooms, and I thought, 'Oh my golly, I'm in my mother's bedroom.' I just couldn't believe it. But I should not have been in that house. Nobody in their right mind would have gone in there."

But there he was, and mainly what he thought was this.

"I want to live forever, but if I have to die, this would be a good place to do it. I'm where I want to be, in my mother's bedroom, in my mother's home place. I really didn't want to leave. I guess that's the closest I've ever been to my mother. It was the most precious moment in my life."

There were actually four levels once, the cellar he jumped over, a first floor that was mostly missing, a second, where he stood now, and an attic, where Bob Small might have hidden himself. There were stairs leading up to the attic, but no attic. The stairs went straight up into the sky, and tempting as it might have been, Sid did not climb them.

"I could have stayed there forever, but looking down that stairway, I knew the longer I stayed, the more dangerous it was going to be getting out."

Also, at some point it dawned on him he was late for lunch. So standing in an empty bedroom with old boards beneath him and the sky right above him, he took out his iPhone and called his sister.

"Beverly, you'll never believe where I'm at."

"Where are you?"

"I'm in your mother's bedroom."

"What? What do you mean?"

"Beverly, I'm upstairs in Mom's home place."

"No you're not."

"Yes I am."

"No you're not."

"But I am."

14

"Number one," Beverly said, "You don't know which room's hers."

"You're right," Sid said. "I don't know which one is hers, but I'm in all three of them."

Beverly never got to number two, and Sid knew it was time to leave.

"I didn't want to leave there. I didn't care about dinner. I didn't know if that house was going to fall down, and I didn't care."

HELEN ARRIVES

Clear Spring, October 1950

The sheriff picked Helen up on July 24 in 1950. It was a Monday and not that hot for July in Washington County. There was big news that day spelled out in bold black print on the front page of the *Hagerstown Morning Herald.*

"Reds Sweep Down West Coast."

These particular Reds were the communist North Koreans, who a month earlier had crossed the 38th parallel that separated communist North Korea from South Korea and very nearly taken the country.

World War II was only five years behind us. Over half a million Americans had recently died. Harry Truman was president at the end of that war. He was president still in 1950. He decided to send the country into war again, and over 33,000 more young American men were about to die far from home in a cold country they knew nothing about.

But that was 7,000 miles away, and Helen wasn't reading the papers. Helen wasn't even talking. She had always been quiet, sort of shy, but also friendly and popular. People liked her, and she liked them. She liked to sit off to the side and watch and listen and laugh. Her mother was the same way. Neither sought lots of attention, or excitement, and both had a sort of calm charisma and natural kindness.

It wasn't the actual sheriff behind the wheel. It was most likely a deputy sheriff named Leister Isanogle. And it's unlikely the deputy sheriff picked Helen up out front of the Starliper home at 221 Main

Street in Clear Spring. It was summer. The seven kids were home. The neighbors would see.

But there was a back yard about 35 feet wide, and at the end of the yard was a big ramshackle barn, two stories tall and older than the house. The barn covered the ground from one side of the yard to the other. Beyond the barn, and past the Starliper property, were nothing but fields that went on forever.

Sid has a picture in his mind of how things went that day. There was a narrow path from the back of the house to the barn, and he sees three women come out of the house and make their way down the path in the morning darkness. Helen's in the middle. Lethean Starliper holds one of Helen's arms. Leila Vance holds the other.

Lethean is Whitey's mom. Leila is Whitey's sister. The women shuffle along. The deputy sheriff's car glides to a stop at the barn. He shuts off his engine. He gets out and opens a back door and helps Helen in. She has a lot of trouble getting into the car, but she smiles. He smiles back. He knows Whitey. He probably knows Helen and has certainly heard of her situation. He holds the other door for Lethean and gently shuts it behind her.

In the back seat, Lethean takes Helen's hand. The sheriff starts his engine and heads slowly south and east out of Clear Spring, out of Washington County, out toward another rural county called Carroll, not that far from Baltimore.

Today they would take I-70, but I-70 wasn't built yet, so they took Route 40 through Hagerstown, probably covering the 70 miles or so in an hour to an hour and a half, depending on how fast the sheriff wanted to get there.

For Lethean, holding Helen's sweating hand in the hot back seat with no air conditioning, the whole thing was a nightmare. She was 64, with a mix of gray and white hair. She wore simple clothes and simple glasses. She was guilt-ridden and heartbroken and filled with worry and doubt.

17

She'd been through a time of near constant trauma. Her husband had just died. Helen had just delivered a baby in the strangest of ways. And three years ago, they'd found cancer in Lethean's colon. They cut it out and rerouted what was left into a bag attached through a hole in her abdomen. They called the procedure a colostomy. They called the hole a stoma.

A nurse brought the bags out to the house and she changed them a few times a week. Lethean was somewhat used to it now and didn't complain much or make any great concessions to the problem.

And through all that, her sickness and surgery and stoma, her husband's death, another baby in their crowded house, she'd also had to watch, in helpless horror, the sad and terrifyingly strange transformation of her son's wife from a loving mother and lovely person into someone completely different. And now they were taking her away from her family and her kids and everything she had ever known.

Helen wore a sundress with stripes that day. The sheriff parked in the lot outside the John Hubner Psychopathic Building near the middle of the Springfield complex. It was a nice building, 35 years old, mostly brick, and arranged like a cross, with a wing heading straight ahead when you walked in and another to the left and another to the right. It was two stories tall, with several wards, a basement, and a big green cupola up top. It was built in 1915 and named for John Hubner, a Baltimore politician who grew up in Bavaria and was widely considered Springfield's founding father.

The hospital opened in 1896 on several hundred acres of land that a farmer and politician named Frank Brown sold to the state for $50,000 at the end of his one term as governor of Maryland. In 1896, they called it "The Second Maryland Hospital for the Insane." Now they called it "Springfield Hospital." Or just Springfield.

Hubner was the central admission point. New patients came in there, where the staff evaluated them and decided where to send them. There was nothing terribly special about the place inside. There was a giant, ornate old mirror in the lobby, but aside from that beautiful mirror, which sits abandoned now in two pieces in the old hospital cannery, the insides of Hubner were institutional and bland. There were hallways and offices, desks and chairs, doctors and nurses and social workers, a wheelchair parked here and there, lead paint on the walls, asbestos in the ceilings and pipes, electric fans blowing it all around in the warm air, procedures to follow, and papers to fill.

A social worker named Beverly Heitmann checked them in. The social workers were mostly women. It was their job to get the papers filled, make the family comfortable, and try to ease the arrivals into their new lives with some compassion and kindness and efficiency.

Helen sat quietly. Lethean read forms and signed them. Finally, a nurse helped Helen into a wheelchair, and Lethean bent over her and said, "Good-bye."

There was probably a hug, a kiss, a last look, tears. And Lethean probably made promises. She would take good care of the kids till Helen got better. Maybe Helen understood. Maybe not. Then Lethean had to break free and watch the nurse roll Helen away, until they turned a corner.

Lethean walked outside and down the steps. Helen was in the hands of strangers now. She was in the system, under the care of the state of Maryland.

The sheriff opened the door and Lethean got in. They rode out through the streets of Springfield. Patients strolled the grounds. Cows barely moved on distant hills. Springfield had once been a great grazing farm owned by a man named George Patterson, whose father, William Patterson, made a lot of money helping arm George Washington during the Revolution.

George Patterson raised beautiful Devon cattle imported from England. He had about 40 slaves. When one escaped in 1848, he offered a $500 reward and made every effort to apprehend him.

He had two dogs, Beauregard and Stonewall Jackson, that accompanied him about his property. He also had a famous sister named Elizabeth, who everyone called "Betsy." She was briefly married to

Napoleon Bonaparte's youngest brother, Jerome. Betsy knew Thomas Jefferson. She knew Aaron Burr and Dolly Madison and the Caton sisters, whose grandfather, Charles Carroll of Carrollton, was the only Catholic to sign the Declaration of Independence.

Her marriage was an international sensation at a time of intense struggle between England and France. Napoleon blockaded the coasts to keep her from landing in Europe. Eventually she was given a hero's welcome in England, where she gave birth to the first American Bonaparte.

There was an amazing story back there, but Lethean didn't know anything about all that. She didn't know that George and his wife Prudence had lost their five-year-old son to a disease they couldn't identify. She didn't know that their daughter Florence had died giving birth and was buried in the cemetery nearby with her dead baby lying on her breast.

She didn't know that Prudence Patterson was Frank Brown's aunt, or that after the death of her husband and daughter, she sold Brown the farm.

None of that mattered. Her mind was fixed on the present and Helen and the six kids and one baby waiting for her back in Clear Spring.

The sheriff drove. Lethean stared. She'd never been to a place like this, so many big beautiful brick buildings, all of it so pretty.

She wondered if she would ever see them again. Or Helen, for that matter.

22878

The patient has been almost mute, but will respond
in her own inarticulate and unintelligible way.

DR. GERTRUDE SONNENFELDT

Although most patients were sent elsewhere, the Hubner Building had south, east, and west wards for housing a limited number. They wheeled Helen down the hall to the south ward. At some point, they gave her a number, posed her with her number, and took a picture.

Helen is up against a wall. She's poorly lit. There's a large shadow behind her head. Nothing covers her shoulders except an inch-wide strap on each.

The picture's cropped above the waist. Helen's hair is short and dark and not styled in any way. It looks plain, parted on the left and combed off her forehead.

If they asked her to smile, she chose not to. She looks a bit angry, perhaps, but probably isn't. She looks young. She looks different, not much like the pictures I've seen from her life before Springfield, the period her doctors referred to as her "pre-morbid state."

In her pre-morbid state, she looked happy. She stood tall and straight and smiled, or she crouched with one or two of her kids. She never looked troubled. There's no hint in those old pictures that someday she would be in a picture like this one, posing for an un-skilled photographer with a poor camera in all her worldly posses-sions with short hair and a number and only 36 years old.

Number 22878.

A small and kindly looking man in his seventies, with silver hair and a necktie, who kept his hands folded behind his back, welcomed 22878 into the system. His name was Gertrude, Dr. Gertrude Sonnenfeldt.

Dr. Sonnenfeldt was required to fill in an admission slip with his impressions of the patient.

He wrote, "On admission here, the patient appears her stated age. She sits quietly on a chair and has an empty smile on her face. Her answers are inarticulate, reminding one of the attempts of a mute to vocalize. When helped to get up from her chair, she follows the suggestion, but walks in goose step fashion. She had wet her dress."

For his initial impression, he wrote, "Organic disease of the central nervous system," and "schizophrenia, catatonic type."

Dr. Sonnenfeldt filled out a standard new patient form referred to as a statistical data sheet. At line 18, the form asked for intellectual make-up. The choices were "idiot, imbecile, moron, borderline, mental defective (degree unspecified), average, above average, and unspecified." The doctor chose "average."

On line 21, under contributing factors, he typed "pregnancy."

Helen arrived in her ward a bit after noon with a slight fever in a fresh change of clothes. The ward nurse described her as "cooperative to regular admission care." She also remarked that her head and body were clean and that Helen was well-nourished and "free of vermin." They treated her for vermin anyway.

They noted a vaccination scar on her left arm and a small scar under her nose and described her body as "very shakey."

They noted that her clothes were of "good" quality and in "fair" condition and that other than what she wore, they found no other articles of any sort on her. They noted that her teeth were her own, that her eyes were brown, that her hair was dark brown, and that she was 5'4" and 115 pounds.

They put her to "bed for observation." She lay quietly on a strange mattress in a strange room filled with troubled strangers in the middle of the afternoon and slept. She got a bit restless around 4 p.m., had a good appetite, and fed herself at 5. Her pulse came down, her breathing slowed, her fever dropped below 100. She lay quietly in bed and slept the rest of the day and all through the night.

By the third day, she was calm and eating well. The fever was gone.

Dr. Sonnenfeldt wrote, "The patient has been almost mute, but will respond in her own inarticulate and unintelligible way. However, she is feeding herself, and while her manners remind one of a little animal, she will eat a goodly amount. She is incontinent part of the time and still walks in this goose-stepping manner. When given a bunch of keys today, she took them and tried to unlock the door."

A Dr. Butterworth conducted a physical and described Helen as "a quiet, friendly woman, who doesn't seem to recognize the significance of this interview."

He said she had trouble making herself understood, because "she speaks quite indistinctly, due apparently to a marked speech defect."

He mentioned "marked tremors of the entire body, including the upper and lower extremities, face, head, and tongue," and that she walked with a "shuffling, stiff gait."

He wrote that Helen was "almost uncommunicative at times," although she "was able to state that she came to the hospital because of 'nerves,' but could explain no further...The patient was friendly and smiling, and seemed to be in contact, at least on a superficial level."

Her blood pressure was high, 170 over 90. She was quite thin, but other than the tremors, the odd walk, and the trouble speaking, the doctor found most other things normal for a woman her age.

HOW HELEN GOT TO SCHOOL

Make sure my wife gets a copy of the book.

SUMMER, 2018—BERNIE HENSON

Sid had three brothers and three sisters, and for reasons none can explain, after their mother left, they seldom spoke of her again. The next time they saw her she was dead, and after the funeral, they went back to their lives and continued to speak very rarely about their mother.

The first one to take an active interest in Helen's past was the oldest, Charlie, who everyone in the family called Sonny. In his later years, Sonny researched the Starlipers in great detail. He looked at land records and deeds and old maps and newspapers. He scoured the Internet. Eventually he produced a short manuscript called *The Seven Starlipers of Clear Spring*.

He also created picture books about the town and the family. But most helpful to me, at least in the beginning, was an incomplete copy of Helen's medical records.

For years, Sonny lived in a house one lot over from Sid. He had all this information, but Sid didn't want anything to do with it. Then came Bob Evans, and soon came Sid pounding at Sonny's door.

First, though, before digging into records and genealogies and all the other things Sonny had found or created, Sid needed to know how Helen got to school. Which meant he had to find the school.

Sonny gave him directions, and shortly after Sid climbed the stairs of the old house, he went looking.

To keep him company, he brought along his sister Betty, who was 77. Betty's husband, Albert, had passed away recently. They'd married young and lived together more than 60 years. There's a picture of her and Albert at the Starliper house in Clear Spring sometime in the late fifties, getting ready for the prom. Albert has a crew cut and reminds me of Buddy Holly. Betty's wearing a big pretty puffy dress. Everything's black and white.

And now Albert was gone, and Betty was lonely. She was sad. Sid came by, and they got to talking about Helen and how she might have gone to school. It was very strange that they had never really talked about their mother before. It was nice doing it now.

Betty remembered a bit more than Sid, but not all that much. She couldn't really answer many of Sid's questions. Her mother had been gone nearly 65 years, and unlike their cousin Shirley, she just couldn't remember back that far.

But as they talked, Sid realized that Betty had been thinking about their mother for years, and mostly keeping it to herself. And not only that, she had some of Helen's things in her basement. She showed him a nice pair of leather toddler shoes, a beautiful set of dishes nicely displayed in a cabinet, a perfectly realistic miniature wood stove that Helen played with, and a ring she used to wear.

Betty had documents, too. There were marriage certificates, death certificates, the memorial program from Helen's funeral, with the names of everyone who came. Betty had been thinking about her mother all these years and hiding all these things and never talking about any of it, and now she was in the car with Sid in search of the old school, but Sonny's directions didn't get them there.

Soon enough they got new directions from a guy named Mike McKee, who we'll meet again, and with their new directions, Sid and Betty went looking one more time. The directions said find Gruber Road and look for a sharp turn. The directions led over railroad tracks and narrow roads with sharp turns and pretty fields and narrow streams gurgling right up to the road, and pretty much to nowhere. Well, not quite nowhere.

There were a few houses. But nothing looked like how Sid expected the school to look. He'd seen a picture of it in black and white, a small building with a roof slanted sharply in both directions, three windows on each wall, a set of rickety wooden stairs leading in, nothing much around, just fields and one tree, not a very nice looking place, one floor, one room, one door, no bathrooms, not much light, and a single teacher paid in pennies to teach kids from miles around in this cold little box of wood.

Eventually, Sid would learn all about that school. He would even find the names of the women who taught there over the years, Anna Miller, Fannie Sterling, Agnes Murphy, Lula Shank, Irene Kerr, Marion Charlton, Mabel Miskell, Julia Shank, Miss Fishel, and Ethel Widmyer, who would sit down and cry afterward if she ever had to punish one of her kids.

Sid pulled into the driveway of one of the few houses. It was a small house, a rancher, and pretty, with trees and all kinds of decorations on the lawn and a mailbox that said Henson. Sid had no idea who Henson was. He politely rapped the door. Nothing happened. He knocked a bit harder. Still nothing. He kept knocking. He figured there was someone named Henson in there, and he was going to flush him out.

And sure enough, the door finally opened, and there stood Henson. Henson's first name was Bernie. Bernie came out, somewhat annoyed at these people pounding on his door. He probably expected some kind of sales pitch, but instead he found a fairly innocent looking guy with his fairly innocent looking sister standing there smiling. Both had white hair and seemed to be in their seventies. There was no sign of Girl Scout cookies or pamphlets about Jesus and Armageddon.

Sid introduced himself with a big smile and told Bernie he was looking for the Sunnyside school. Bernie raised his arm and pointed.

"See that house right there? That house right there is the Sunnyside school."

And just like that, Sid had found Helen's school. Except now it was a house. It still had the roof from its schoolhouse days. Sid noticed that someone had added an addition, making it larger than the old school, but smaller than the typical house. He noticed a hole they'd patched when they relocated the chimney.

His mom had probably been in there over a thousand times, back when men he knew nothing about, men like Warren G. Harding and Calvin Coolidge, were Presidents of the United States, back after the First World War ended and the Roaring Twenties arrived.

And Helen sat right over there in that old building in some old desk with her pencils and books and a pen she dipped into a well for ink. There was a woodstove and wooden floors and a blackboard smeared with erased chalk and one teacher for all the grades. And sometimes Helen shivered in there and sometimes it was hot and sometimes the teacher sent her out to clap erasers, and she would stand not a hundred yards from where Sid stood now, right by that small house, holding her arms straight out from her face, squinting, turning her head, clapping the erasers, a big cloud of chalk blowing back and dusting her clothes and hair and sticking in her eyelashes. And no doubt she laughed.

Right over there she would have stood. They could have walked across the grass to one another in a matter of seconds, except she stood there in 1924, and Sid stood there in 2016.

It turns out Bernie shared Sid's interest in the school. He went back into his house and came out with a piece of old wood, shaped something like a very short oar, or maybe an overgrown paddle of some sort. It had a flat surface and a nice handle but didn't seem ideally suited to any sport Sid knew.

When Bernie was a kid, they were remodeling the school, and one day he wandered over and found the thing under the floor. He scrawled something on the handle on a big piece of white tape.

"Found By B.W. Henson JR. '1962' Sunnyside School House, Big Spring, MD – Homeplace, Ball Bat or Paddle."

Sid held the thing. Then Betty held it. They all laughed and tried to figure out what it was. It seemed awfully big for an instrument of punishment and certainly not something Ethel Widmyer would ever use. It was awfully small for an oar, and it certainly wasn't a baseball bat. The handle was round, but the paddle was flat.

Sid gave it back to Bernie. And from that point on they were friends. Sid would visit. They would do research together and speculate about the school and how Helen got there. Sid was pretty sure the Smalls never had a horse. And she didn't take the bus, because Sid found an article from the September 6, 1930, *Hagerstown Morning Herald*, a couple years after Helen graduated, and it said, "The school bus leaving Charlton at 8:15 every morning made its maiden trip September 2 with Millard Kretzer as driver and seventeen happy boys and girls."

Too late for Helen. Eventually, they convinced themselves she walked. There was a long walk, about a mile and a half, and a short walk about half as long. The long way stuck to the streets. The short way cut straight across a field in front of Helen's house. The only problem with the short way was that right before the field's end, just short of the school, there was a brook too difficult to cross.

Then one day Sid found another *Herald* article from 1926 that helped clear things up.

"The heavy rains have taken away the bridge on which several children from Two Locks cross while coming to school. This bridge was constructed only a few months ago by the patrons in the place of the old one which was destroyed by the high water in the summer."

In 1926, Helen would have been 13 and probably in her last year. It's quite likely she was one of the kids from Two Locks who crossed the bridge until it washed out, then crossed it again, when they built another, until that washed out.

So, they decided. Helen walked. When the bridge was in, she walked three-quarters of a mile across a field and over a stream. And when the bridge was out, she went the long way.

The school closed in 1940. The county sold it to Frank C. Zimmerman for $200, and from then on, the kids from Two Locks, and all the other kids from the little homes that dotted the countryside, were bused to school in Clear Spring.

Sid had the answer to his first big question. And he continued to visit his new friend. Then one day, well over a year since their first meeting, Sid sent me a photo. He's sitting in a chair in Bernie's house. It's July of 2018. Sid's wearing a black baseball cap that says, "Chevrolet." He's holding Bernie's paddle with two hands.

Bernie's lying on a bed. He's thin with black hair and big glasses. Bernie's holding the paddle, too, and smiling a bit, but not as much as Sid's smiling. There's a tube running across Bernie's chest and up into his nose.

One day Sid came to visit, and they were wheeling Bernie out to an ambulance. And then, about two weeks after Sid sent me the picture, he sent me a text.

"Jack, Bernie passed away last night."

Sid and his daughter, Beth, got to visit him a couple days before the end. By now Bernie considered Sid one of his best friends. He had some last words for Sid.

"Make sure my wife gets a copy of the book."

And then he gave Sid the paddle he found under the schoolroom floor in 1962.

THE BABY WHO DIDN'T CRY

I can still see her laying there in the bed with the baby all by herself. I'll never forget. I just felt so sorry for her.

HARRIET CLOPPER, 2018

Clear Spring, April 1949

Several people mentioned in this story died while I wrote it. Bernie was the second. The first was Sid's brother Sonny (Charlie), who died about a month before Bernie. Sonny was born on November 2, 1937. He excelled at school and soccer, but his passion was something called Soap Box Derby. He built his own cars out of wood and roller skate wheels and raced downhill in a helmet. with gravity for power, bouncing, and gripping the wheel, and trying to get to the bottom faster than anyone else.

In July of 1950 when he was 13, he even made the paper as one of three Clear Spring boys who would be competing in Hagerstown that weekend for a trip to the championships in Akron, Ohio. He didn't make it, though, and 11 days later, his mother left for Springfield. It's not likely she saw Sonny's big race.

Sonny wore glasses. He had blonde hair with some waves in it. There's a picture from 1962. He's wearing a T-shirt and smiling with his arm around Lethean. She's got a big smile and an arm around his waist. Her head barely reaches his shoulder.

After high school, Sonny went to community college in Hagerstown and then on to the University of Maryland. He majored in History and became an expert on World War II. He met a girl named Lois, and they were married and had two daughters. He joined the navy in 1960 and spent nine years as a navy officer, serving on seven different aircraft carriers.

By December of 1967, during the peak of the Vietnam war, he was a lieutenant and a photographic air intelligence officer on the USS Coral Sea, an aircraft carrier in the Gulf of Tonkin off the coast of North Vietnam.

Eventually, he left the navy and became head of personnel at the National Academy of Science in downtown D.C. and worked there for many years, despite a terrible four-hour daily commute.

The first thing I did, even before heading out to Clear Spring or talking at length with Sid, was to look at the medical records Sonny passed along. The records originated on microfilm. The paper was gray. A lot of the text was handwritten and hard to read, the records seemed incomplete, and they were definitely out of order, and no matter how hard I tried, I couldn't quite get them back in order.

Things were missing. The numbering was confusing. Sid was trying to get a new set. But one thing I was able to piece together from Sonny's gray records was the unusual story of Patsy Starliper's birth. By the time it happened, Helen was 35, already had six children, and had been living with the Starlipers a bit over 10 years.

She had her first five all in a row between 1937 and 1943— Sonny, Beverly, Betty, Bob, and Sid. After Sid, there was a break, and then Dave came along in September 1947. By late summer of 1948, Helen was pregnant again and due the following May. The timing was terrible.

About three months before Helen's due date, in February of '49, Lethean's husband, Sam, felt something come over him. They'd been married over 40 years and raised six kids. He was 75. He got into his bed. He made out a will on February 7 and died on March 6. It was his heart.

And there was something else going on, too, something with Helen. She wasn't right, and there's a good chance she hadn't been during her last pregnancy, or even before that. She tried keeping things to herself, but they were getting worse, and eventually there was no way to hide them. For the longest time, she was just tired, persistently tired in an overwhelming way.

Now she had trouble walking. First, she dragged a leg. Soon, she shuffled along nervously, struggling to keep her balance. And she was moody, depressed, detached, and slowly losing touch with her life, her kids, her responsibilities.

The family doctor noticed her walk, and probably several other odd and worrisome symptoms, and suggested she have the baby in the hospital. He also wanted her sterilized while there. He seemed to think her problems might have something to do with all those babies coming one after another, and sterilization seemed like the best way to put an end to it. Apparently, Dr. Sonnenfeldt suspected something similar and noted "pregnancy" in the hospital records as a possible contributing factor.

About eight months into her pregnancy and not long after the family doctor mentioned the hospital, Helen sent Sonny out to the store. Sonny was smart and mature for his age, but she sent him to buy something he probably didn't know anything about.

It's possible she sent Sonny because she didn't want any of the adults in the family to know what she was doing. Whatever the case, he came home with a box of sanitary napkins. Helen opened them and put them aside near her bed. Lethean noticed but didn't say anything and didn't know what to make of it.

The next night, on April 13, 1949, a month before the baby was due, Helen lay in bed, as usual. Most likely, Whitey was out drinking. Most likely, he came home late and found her sleeping, or pretending. He fell asleep beside her. Bob, Dave, and Sid slept in their bed just a foot or so away.

And somehow, with four other people in the room, without waking any of them, Helen had a baby. If she moaned or cried, no one heard. If the baby cried, no one heard. No one woke up. In the morning, Whitey thought he felt Helen's knees shaking. He opened his eyes and found Helen and his seventh child lying in the bed beside him.

Later that day, a good friend of Whitey's oldest sister, Leila, stopped by. Her name was Harriet Clopper. She was a frequent visitor who would just walk right in. She called Lethean "Stoppy."

Harriet turned 100 while I wrote this. When she was much younger, she ran a bar with her husband. They had a big shuffleboard downstairs, and Whitey used to drink there. They had a very pretty daughter. Sid had a crush on her and would hang out with her in her room above the bar.

And later, for years, Harriet worked at the Clear Spring McDonalds right behind the old Starliper house. She worked there into her nineties and at one point was the oldest McDonald's worker in the world.

Harriet found Helen alone that day on a bed with her baby. Helen smiled at Harriet. Harriet smiled back and said, "hello," and that was all. They didn't talk. Helen didn't invite Harriet over to look at the baby.

Harriet was a teenager then, and now, more than 85 years later, she says, "I can still see her laying there in the bed with the baby all by herself. I'll never forget. I just felt so sorry for her."

The baby was fine and healthy. They named her Patricia.

DAM 5

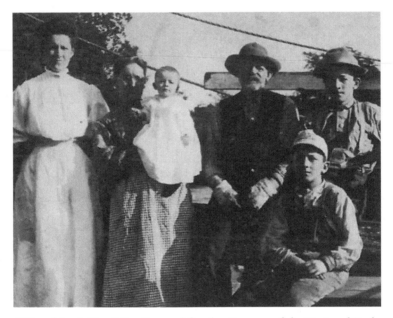

"Guard Lock Dan" Sterling and family. *Courtesy of the National Park Service, C&O Canal NHP.*

C&O Canal, 1903

When I met Sid, I didn't know anything about the C&O Canal. It was something I might have heard of, a bike path on an abandoned canal somewhere in Western Maryland. I thought it sounded boring. But actually, the canal isn't boring at all. In its day, it was a technological marvel, doomed and surpassed by more practical technology, but still, an amazing achievement.

The idea was to build a waterway along the Potomac River connecting the Chesapeake Bay to the Ohio River. John Quincy Adams, the sixth President and son of the second, was there at its inception on July 4, 1828, to turn over a spade of dirt and initiate decades of constant struggle.

The canal builders, officially the C&O Canal Company, were in a race with the B&O Railroad, which had similar goals and many advantages and got to work at the same time. This was hard manual labor. Picks and shovels and a dangerous explosive called black powder. (Dynamite wouldn't come along until the late 1860s.) This was carving a waterway through miles of ancient rock and earth, foot by foot, inch by inch, man against nature in a time when man had only crude tools at his disposal.

There weren't enough locals willing to do the work. The canal company advertised in Europe and attracted indentured laborers with the promise of three meals a day, ample quantities of meat, vegetables, and whiskey, and about ten dollars a month. Mostly, it was the Irish who came, single men, desperate sorts, willing to work for low wages under terrible conditions. Others came from England and Wales and Germany.

The weather was hot and humid. Or freezing cold. There were legal disputes with the B&O over land rights. There were supply shortages. There were constant labor shortages. There were labor riots. The Irish fought among themselves with fists and knives and the various tools at their disposal. Sometimes guns. They fought the English. They fought the Germans. They fought mosquitos and terrible disease.

They drank tremendous amounts of liquor. They lived in damp, dirty, makeshift, and unsanitary shanties they built themselves, then took down, then built again, as they made their slow progress alongside the river.

There were deadly bouts of cholera, a wretched disease, caused by toxic bacteria. In 1832, the so-called Asiatic cholera moved down from Montreal and into the canal at Harper's Ferry. The workers called it the "pestilence." It caused terrible diarrhea and vomiting, massive dehydration, and physical pain.

Death came fast, but not fast enough. Great numbers of Irish died far from home. Some are buried in unmarked graves along the Potomac. Many who didn't die got out of there fast.

But they came back, or were replaced, and work went on. They completed the canal in sections. Once a section was ready, they opened it. The first section, connecting Georgetown in Washington, D.C., to Seneca, Maryland, covered about 25 miles and took three years to build. By the time they reached Cumberland, Maryland, in 1850, about halfway to their original goal, they were eight years behind the railroad and far behind their own schedule.

They stopped. They had built a canal 184.5 miles long, connecting Cumberland, Maryland, and Washington, D.C. They thought the whole project would take three years. It took 22 to get halfway.

During those 22 years, they built lift locks, guard locks, and lockhouses. They built 11 stone aqueducts to carry the canal over streams. They built dams along the river to supply water for the canal. They clawed a 3,100-foot tunnel through a mountain. They called it the Paw Paw Tunnel. It was long, narrow, dark, and spooky. It could only accommodate one boat heading in one direction at a time. It took 14 years to build.

The canal ran alongside the north bank of the Potomac, but it was nothing like a river or stream or any naturally occurring body of water. A canal boat starting at sea level at Georgetown would complete its journey 610 feet above sea level at Cumberland, Maryland. They were actually moving boats from lower elevations to higher elevations.

Which is what the lift locks were for. There were 77. On its way up to Cumberland, a mostly empty canal boat would enter each lock at one level, water would fill the lock, the boat would rise with the water, then leave the lock at a new elevation. So, by traveling from lock to lock, and entering and exiting the locks at progressively higher levels, the boats could use water to move uphill. They called each stretch of canal between a pair of locks a "level." Levels could be quite short or several miles long.

Coming the other way through the canal, boats filled with cargo, mostly coal from the Alleghenies, would do the opposite, moving from higher elevations to lower elevations through the locks. Only now they were heavy and low in the water with 120 tons of coal. They had a small current behind them, moving about two miles an hour.

The boats had no means of powering themselves, no engines, sails, oars, just that moderate current to move them along, and only when loaded up and heading south toward Georgetown. Mainly, they were powered by mules, two at a time attached to the boats by thick rope. The mules and the boys and girls who guided them travelled down a path 12 feet wide called the towpath. The towpath ran between the canal and the river.

The canal itself was six feet deep. It was 60 feet wide at most points, with exceptions, like the Paw Paw Tunnel. All along it lived lockkeepers and their families in homes built by the canal company. The lockkeepers got a house, a small salary paid monthly, about $22 in 1916 and about $35 in 1924, and an acre of land to grow things. In return, they operated the machinery to let the boats in and drain and fill the locks so the boats could move up or down to the next level.

There was a small cabin of sorts down by the lock, where the lockkeeper could stay out of the rain, or sun, or get a bit of warmth in winter.

It was an all-day job. When a canal boat approached a lock, someone on board blasted a few warning notes on a horn, and whether it was 5 a.m. or midnight, someone else had to come out and let the boat through. Usually the lockkeeper. But it might be his wife, or a son, or a daughter.

The typical lockhouse had three floors. It had two bedrooms upstairs, two rooms down below, a two-room cellar with dirt floors, and several fireplaces. By today's standards they were primitive, but by the standards of the time, they were relatively comfortable.

The boat operators had the rougher lives. They actually lived on their skinny 90-foot-long boats at least eight months a year with four mules and, often, entire families. Some lived on their boats year-round.

They stored food on the boats. They used kerosene and corncobs to set coal burning in a small cookstove. They scrubbed their laundry on deck on washboards over big pots of hot water, then poured the water into the canal. They ran clotheslines from one end of their boats to the other. They heated irons on cookstoves to press their clothes. They poured food waste into the canal. They used chamber pots and dumped them into the canal.

They slept in narrow bunks. Small children often wore harnesses strapped to the cabin on the boat to keep them from falling off into the water.

During its best years in the 1870s, there were some 500 canal boats, sometimes packed like cars on a highway, moving tons of coal from Cumberland to Washington, thousands of men, women, children, and mules heading up and down that long thin strip of water.

There were seven dams. Dam 5 spanned the river from Maryland to Virginia. (West Virginia wasn't established until 1853.) The dam opened in 1835. Because of the rock cliffs at that point along the Maryland shore, the canal builders couldn't extend the canal through, so at Dam 5 the boats had to go out into the river.

These breaks in the canal, where the boats were forced to travel temporarily through the Potomac, were called "slackwaters." There were only two. The one near Dam 5 was about half a mile long and called "Little Slackwater."

A boat heading back up toward Cumberland, which would be mostly empty, or what they called "light," would go out into the river at Dam 5 through something called a guard lock, which also controlled the flow of water from the river into the canal, then travel that half mile, and reenter the canal at Lock 45. Since Lock 46 followed almost immediately after 45, they called the area Two Locks. And it was in that small stretch of concrete towpath, rock cliffs, and half mile or so of land that Helen's family lived and grew and died.

Mary Kate Sterling was born in 1847. She was one of several children, with five older brothers and one older sister. Everyone called her Kate. Her father, Samuel Sterling, was born in 1810. In 1833, for $1500, about $31,000 in today's money, Samuel's father sold him just about all a young man would need to get started in the business of farming.

That included a farm wagon, two plows, four sets of wagon gear, four mares, three colts, a white cow, a black and white cow, a white bull, a black bull, and as the official document of sale states, a "negro woman about thirty five years old, one negro girl about seven years old," and four other young "negroes," ranging between four and thirteen.

In other words, when Kate's father began his career as a farmer in Williamsport, Maryland, he was 23 and the owner of seven horses, four cows, and six people. He married Ellen Williams in 1837, and they began turning out young Sterlings.

The slaves were gone by 1847, when Kate came along, and when the Civil War began in 1861, three of Kate's brothers fought for the Union. Two others were turned away.

Kate's oldest brother, John Sterling, was the first member of the family to set up in the area between Dam 5 and Two Locks. He was also the first to take fire during the war, when in December of 1861, the Confederates took to shooting across the river at his farm.

They weren't actually shooting at him. They were shooting at his barn, where several members of the 13th Massachusetts Infantry regiment were trying to sleep. The soldiers were there to defend the dam, which Stonewall Jackson was trying to blow up, or otherwise subvert, to keep coal out of Washington.

Jackson's men did some damage, but never managed to destroy the dam. They did manage to hit John Sterling's barn with cannon fire. The barn burst into flames, and not long after that, John Sterling moved with his family to Iowa and never took part in the war.

The three brothers who did enlist, George, Henry, and Samuel B., all fought. George Sterling fought at Gettysburg with the first Maryland Cavalry. He took a bullet in the knee at the battle of Appomattox Court House in 1865, just hours before Robert E. Lee gave up the fight. When George died in 1902, he still had that bullet in his leg and was buried in his old uniform under an America flag.

Of the three brothers, it was Samuel B. who took the most bold and risky action. He deserted. His father was sick and debilitated, and the family back home was destitute, with several children and all the older sons gone. Samuel went home, and soon after, in 1865, his father died in Clear Spring at 56.

Kate was about 17 when her father died. Three years later, she married a veteran of the war named Robert Harry Small. Robert's father was a tailor. Robert was a shoemaker and a musician. During the war, he served as the leader of a popular regimental band and was well known in the Clear Spring area.

Robert was born in 1831. He was 16 years older than Kate, who was 20 when she married him. They had a son in 1868 and named him Harry Sterling Small. They lived in dwelling number 90 in Clear Spring. Living with Robert, Kate, and young Harry was Robert's sister, Ann V. Reid, who was just over 35 and had already lost two husbands.

On September 22 of 1877, Robert overdosed on laudanum. Or maybe chloroform. The papers called it suicide, and most likely it was, but the papers weren't terribly reliable. They disagreed on various basic details, including his age, how many children he had, and whether it was laudanum or chloroform that killed him. They couldn't even seem to decide whether his name was Robert Harry, Robert Harvey, or just Harvey.

But these are facts. Robert was dead. Kate was 30 and a widow.

I'm not sure what happened to Robert's sister Ann at that point, but Kate took young Harry and moved back home with her mother. Kate worked as a seamstress. Harry grew up in Clear Spring with his mother, his grandmother, and Kate's youngest brothers, Daniel and Joseph.

Daniel was in his twenties when Kate showed up with her son. During the war, Daniel had walked 30 miles from Williamsport to Frederick to enlist in the Union army, but they sent him home. Daniel was brave, but he was also 14, and the war was just about over.

Now Daniel was a boatman on the canal. So was his brother, Joseph. And they probably took their young nephew Harry out on the water from time to time. Harry attended the local schools through seventh grade and went to work at a very young age to help support the family. He's listed in the 1880 census as an 11-year-old farmer. Somewhere along the line, he learned carpentry.

In 1884, Kate remarried, this time to Dr. Scott Gardner, also of Clear Spring. Dr. Gardner was 30. She was 37. By 1889, Scott Gardner was dead, and Kate was 42 and a widow again.

A year after his mother lost her second husband, Harry Small found a wife, a likable Clear Spring girl named Annie Shupp. Harry and Annie were both 22 and born in 1868. Annie's parents were Mennonite farmers, who'd moved to Clear Spring from Lancaster, Pennsylvania, the so-called Pennsylvania Dutch Country.

THE NEIGHBORHOOD

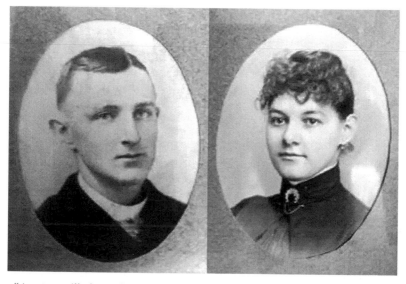

"Annie, we'll always be together." Young Harry Small and Annie Shupp. In the end, she lived nine years without him.

In 1894, over 30 years after Confederate troops blew up their brother's barn, Kate's brother Daniel Sterling moved into the lockhouse at Dam 5. Daniel was married now and brought along a wife and three children.

For the next 25 years, Daniel and his family would be the keepers of the dam and the guard lock that controlled the flow of water from the river into the canal. The guard lock also controlled the passage of canal boats out into the river.

In 1896, two years after Daniel's family moved into the lockhouse, Harry Small's aunt, Ann V. Reid, bought a property on a cliff staring out over the slackwater on the Potomac, about halfway between Dam 5, where canal boats went out into the river, and Lock 45, where they reentered the canal. She paid $200.

Kate was her sister-in-law. Harry was her nephew. Soon, Harry, his wife Annie, and their three kids moved into the house with Harry's aunt. By 1903, there were five kids, due to the arrival of twins named Earl and Esther. At that point, his aunt sold her land and her home to Harry for two dollars, as long as he would let her live there.

Harry was happy to make the deal. He was about 35 now, balding, creative, argumentative, eccentric. Sid's cousin Shirley laughs a happy musical laugh, when she remembers her great grandfather.

"Grandpa Small was a funny old fella. He was grouchy just to be grouchy. He used to get on my great grandma. He'd aggravate her. They wore long dresses then, and she would have her apron on and she would just fold that apron up around her arm and she would go outside. She would go out in the garden. She'd find some excuse to get away from him.

"He used to sit back behind the stove. There was a bench that came from the chimney over to the pie safe. It was just big enough for one person to sit back there. In those days in those houses they all had a place behind the stove, a little chimney corner or whatever. He'd sit back there with his glasses on, reading the Bible, and he'd eat ice cream and put pepper on it, and then he'd go out and get them all worked up at the store."

The store was a short stroll down the towpath at Lock 46. Henry Tedrick opened it in 1894. He did good business. He rented out mules. He sold things in quantity—kegs of sugar and nails and molasses, barrels of coal and oil, cheese in round blocks, large quantities of flour, salt, and buckwheat. And groceries, too, and feed.

He sold long black licorice. He sold penny candy. He sold peanuts for two cents a bag. For three cents a bottle, he sold a new drink called Coca-Cola that was originally concocted by a pharmacist and came with a bit of cocaine in it. He sold something called snappy cheese that a man named Wilson Rhodes told Sid about many years later. Wilson was a friend of the Starliper family, a war hero, and member of a tank battalion, who was born in 1917, lived 99 years, and never forgot snappy cheese.

The store was a friendly place. It carried those basic necessities. It carried cigarettes and newspapers. It was the post office and the telegraph office. And since there wasn't much else around, the store was a hangout where people could gossip and smoke their pipes and argue about politics. And that's where Harry went for fun.

Harry was smart with a great memory and a head full of facts. He ran a clever and complex operation, pursued self-sufficiency, and had lots of nice stuff in his house, but no one knows where, or how, he got it. Shirley thinks he also had money in the bank, but she doesn't know how much or how he got that, either.

He certainly never had any sort of high-paying job. In one census he's listed as a quarry worker. In others he's a laborer or a carpenter. Being a carpenter on a canal made mostly of wood was probably a good thing. The canal broke a lot. Sometimes in small ways, often in catastrophic. And someone had to put it back together. But that didn't seem like the road to riches.

Since the Smalls now had five children, and the Sterlings had added another, there were, in that quarter-mile stretch between the lockhouse at Dam 5 and the house up on the cliffs where the Smalls lived, at least 15 Sterlings and Smalls, brothers, sisters, cousins, aunts, uncles, mothers, fathers, all within a short walk on the towpath along the river.

It was nice arrangement, at least for Harry, and assuming that his wife, Annie, was okay living with Harry's aunt and only a few minutes from all those Sterlings, it was nice for her, too. She was a good-natured sort, and had to be, because Harry was a bit of a pest and took great joy in teasing her.

Shirley says, "Poor grandma Small was just a tiny little thing. Quiet and just smiling all the time. I remember the rain barrel at the corner of the house. She used to go out there and get water and water her flowers with that. And we'd get out there and mess with the water and she'd say, 'Don't waste the water, don't waste the water.'"

Harry loved her, too. Once on a stroll down to the river, one of his granddaughters noticed Harry and Annie sitting on a log holding hands. She heard him say, "Annie, we'll always be together."

But there were things working against them. They were stalked by bad luck and tragedy. Sometimes disaster just missed them. Sometimes it didn't miss them, in ways that are almost impossible to believe.

One of the near misses took place in 1903, when Harry's youngest daughter, Esther, caught fire. She was five. She was running around in one of her mom's dresses, when she got too close to a woodstove and was immediately swallowed in flames. She screamed. Annie ran from another room and doused Esther from a bucket of water and saved her life.

A SLENDER THREAD

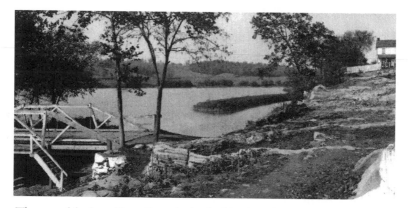

The guard lock at Dam 5, with the lockhouse where the Sterlings lived in the distance. *Courtesy of the National Park Service, C&O Canal NHP.*

The details of the affair obtained from the scene by a Mail reporter constitute a chapter of thrilling facts showing upon what a slender thread human life hangs.

THE DAILY MAIL, MAY 8, 1903

Dam 5, May 1903

The same year that Esther caught fire, on May 1, 1903, the Sterlings at Dam 5 were deeply involved in one of the canal's great tragedies. It was a Friday morning about 10. Ralph and Harry Newkirk, whose father had taken over the Two Locks store, were on the Sterling's land that day, plowing a field with a horse. Ralph was 16. Harry was 18, and they saw it at about the same time, a canal boat heading out into the river beyond the dam against a strong wind.

On board were Captain Joseph Kime, his wife, and their daughters. Clara was 10. Mary was 7. There were also two mules on board, including one who was blind. The other mules were on the towpath, attached to the boat by a rope. Guiding the mules was an inexperienced mule boy.

According to the *Hagerstown Daily Mail*, it was "boat number 6 of the Canal Towage Company's fleet," coming up from Williamsport. There had been a storm the night before. The winds were still strong. The river ran fast toward the dam, and as the mule boy on the towpath led the boat out into the river against the current, a gust of wind grabbed it. The rope between the boat and the mules strained.

Harry Newkirk ran from the Sterling's field toward the boat. Years later, perhaps out of modesty, he would claim he merely wanted a ride up the river to home, which seems awfully foolish. It seems more likely he was trying to help the captain, but whatever his motives, he leaped, and barely made it onto the boat.

The boat was light. The wind and current working against it were heavy. The weight of Harry Newkirk made no difference. From the porch of the house, Daniel Sterling's daughter Mary, and his wife, Virginia, watched.

At the guard lock the boat had just passed through, Daniel Sterling also watched. The guard lock was a complicated thing that a boat had to go through to get out into the river. Daniel was in charge of the lock. He was 52 and had been keeper of that lock nearly 10 years now.

Along the C&O, they called him "Guard Lock Dan," or "Lockkeeper Dan." Daniel knew the river and the dam and understood that conditions, which were always dangerous at that point, were treacherous now.

He warned the captain that his towline appeared frayed and probably wouldn't be up to the job. The captain ignored him. He told the captain that two other boats had failed to navigate out into the river in the storm and had narrowly averted disaster, one on Thursday night, and one earlier that morning. But the captain wasn't listening.

Daniel tried the captain's wife. He asked her to bring down her girls. It was only a half mile up the towpath to Lock 45, a short walk to safety. They could meet the captain there when he came in off the river. Mrs. Kime laughed a bit, and half joking, said she'd stay on the boat with her girls and the "old man," and if it came to it, they would all drown together.

And so, the family went out into the water against the current and the wind. On the towpath, the mules pulled. The mule boy struggled. The dam roared behind the boat. Captain Kime held the tiller and steered against the wind. Then came a loud crack. Either the rope had snapped, or the mule boy cut it to prevent the mules from being pulled into the river. In either case, the boat swirled out deeper and backward toward the dam. The mule boy panicked and ran and was never seen again.

Daniel Sterling grabbed a skiff. Ralph Newkirk jumped in with him. They headed out toward the boat. They tried to reach its rope, but the boat was out too far and moving too fast. And as Mary and Virginia watched from the lockhouse, the boat rolled over the dam, out of sight, and down 20 feet into the rocks and water below, with a tremendous crash. Virginia Sterling fainted.

The boat landed on its side. The girls and the mother in the main cabin were thrown from one side of the boat to the other. Mary washed out the cabin window. Her sister Clara slammed against the wall. Then the family's stove slammed her. Her leg broke, and then, she, too, was flushed out into the roaring foam.

Once it hit the bottom of the waterfall, the boat quickly righted itself and hurled Captain Kime into the air. He landed on deck, sprawled out, unmoving, and apparently dead.

Harry Newkirk was in the river. Somehow, he got hold of the boat's rudder blade. The mother stuck her head out of a hole in the cabin and shouted to Harry. Had he seen her girls? His teeth were broken. Blood poured out his mouth. He hadn't seen her girls.

Meanwhile Dan Sterling and Ralph Newkirk had abandoned their first skiff, grabbed another below the falls, and headed to the rescue. They pulled Harry aboard. Then the captain. They rescued Mrs. Kime and her daughter, Clara. But the other daughter was gone.

Daniel and his wife, Virginia, along with Ralph Newkirk and Mary Sterling, helped the wounded captain, his wife, their injured daughter, and the drenched and exhausted Harry Newkirk into the lockhouse. They wrapped them in blankets and cleaned them up. They put them in bed.

A boy named Tedrick grabbed a horse and galloped along the towpath toward Williamsport. Soon a doctor arrived.

A few days later they found the captain's drowned daughter. A short time after that the captain died, as they tried to move him from the lockhouse to the hospital. The mother and daughter with her broken leg were taken away, most likely destitute.

Daniel's daughter Mary would never forget that day. Even in 1973 as an old woman named Mary Mouse sitting with an equally aged Harry Newkirk, and a popular reporter for the Hagerstown Daily Mail named Ora Ann Ernst, she could call it all clearly to mind.

In the May 19th issue of the paper, Ernst wrote, "Vivid yet to her are the sunsets over the dam as seen from the porch of her home and dramatic is her mind's picture of the break-up of ice on the river, with huge pieces going over the falls.

"She is still amazed by the remembered phenomenon of large trees going over the dam, being caught in the powerful undertow that threw them back to the falls again and again for as long as four days, and left them denuded of all limbs and branches."

But nothing compared to the memory of Captain Kime's boat going over the side with a huge booming crash, like one of those trees the river would strip clean.

THE RAM

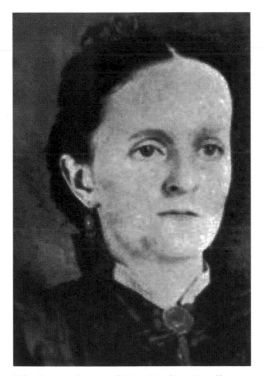

The haunted eyes of Kate Sterling Small
Gardner. Date unknown.

It was a terrible event, the little girl washing away, her father dying in
pain and guilt and fear with broken ribs and a broken heart. No
doubt it was big news all along the canal and certainly in the neigh-
borhood of Harry Small, Daniel Sterling, and the Two Locks store.

But it didn't strike the Smalls and the Sterlings directly, no matter how much it excited and upset them.

At this point in Harry's house, there were Harry, Annie, five children, and Ann Reid. I've seen her name as Ann, Annie, and Anna. We'll go with Ann to distinguish her from Harry's wife, Annie.

Ann was born in 1834. Her first husband died young. Then she married a soldier named Francis C. Reid. Francis Reid fought with the Union for three years. He survived the war but died a short time later.

By her mid-thirties, Ann was a widow twice and living with her brother Robert, her sister-in-law Kate, and young Harry. Then her brother took poison. Her sister-in-law and nephew moved in with Kate's mother, and Ann was alone for a while.

Eventually, she bought her home along the canal. She invited her nephew and his family in. And she had a family. I'm sure it's no coincidence that she bought a home a short walk from Kate Sterling's brother. Kate also lived somewhere close by.

Ann Reid was a small person. I've seen a poorly copied picture of her when she was younger, although I can't say how young. She had big cheeks and big happy eyes and an eager face. She's not actually smiling, but she radiates friendliness, intelligence, and humor. It's like she's looking out at life and can't wait to get started. You can't look at that picture without thinking, this is a person who deserves a happy life.

It could have been a very lonely one, with two husbands gone so young. But she had Harry and Annie and all their kids and all those Sterlings just up the towpath. Then one morning in 1905, two years after Captain Kime and his family washed over the dam, Harry's aunt went for a walk. She probably did that all the time. She said she had business to tend to and would be back that afternoon.

There wasn't all that much around, just a few trees, lots of fields, the skinny road that ran up from the dam and by the house, and somewhere out there, a ram.

No one thinks of sheep as violent animals, but the typical ram weighs over 300 pounds, can run 25 miles an hour, and has horns that might grow to 30 inches long. They don't seem particularly smart. When a couple get together, they like to charge each other and bang heads.

At some point, Ann saw the ram. At some point, she realized that the ram saw her. And then she ran. At least that's what one account says. But there were no witnesses.

Four hours after Ann left the house, a child found her in the grass. She was on her back, bleeding from over a dozen wounds. Her dress was shredded. Her face was mutilated. Great hunks of hair were ripped from her head. In the distance stood the ram with blood on its face and hair in its horns.

Her heart was beating. They carried her home. They put her in bed. She died on her 71st birthday.

A year later, Kate died, just short of 60, in the house nearby where she lived. Like Ann Reid, Kate had also lost two husbands. And I've seen a picture of her, too, but further along than the picture of Ann, or so it seems. Kate's mouth is a straight thin line. Her eyes look off from the camera. She shows no awareness of its presence. Her forehead is high, her hair is pulled back and held in place by a barrette of some sort. She's wearing dangling earrings, a nice dress, and a broach at her neck.

It seems she prepared well for the photo, but there's not a trace of joy on her face. There's nothing resembling a smile. Her face is a blank. It's similar to a look I would see in another picture on another face taken many years later of Sid's sister Patsy.

Harry wasn't 40 yet. Both his parents had died young. His aunt had been mauled by a sheep. His youngest daughter had nearly burned to death. And the same year that his mother died, his wife had another baby. They named him Harry Randolph Small.

Time moved. The river spilled over the dam. The mules pulled. The boats, heavy with coal from the mountains, slipped by beneath the rocks in Harry Small's backyard.

The great European powers continued to arm for a war no one really wanted. And it was 1913.

THE BABY

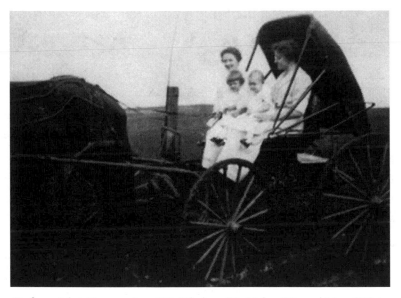

(Left to right) Devona (age 23), Thelma (2), Helen (1), and Nan (21) in 1914. Devona and Nan are Helen's sisters. Helen is Thelma's aunt.

Two Locks, 1913

Two Locks was beautiful and isolated, with just a few narrow roads and nothing much around except farmland. Cars were scarce. There were no lightbulbs. There were no streetlamps. It was pitch black at night. Trains whistled in the distance and the stars went on forever.

They heated with wood and coal. There was a hole in the foundation where Harry shoveled coal down into the cellar. They had plenty of heat, but there was no refrigerator. There was no electricity at all, for that matter. There was no indoor plumbing. The only thing remotely modern was an amazing invention that carried human voices on wire and came to the canal in 1879 for the convenience of the Canal Company.

It was one of the first telephone systems in Maryland. It went from Georgetown to Cumberland on miles of wire strung from poles made from chestnut trees, 30 poles per mile, 25 feet high, 5,665 of them. At first, they installed 46 phones, and Daniel Sterling's brother, Samuel B. Sterling, who once left the army to save his family, got one. Samuel worked out of a maintenance shed on the canal and one of the phones went to "Sterling's Shanty," making Harry's uncle Sam one of the first men in Maryland, and the country, with a telephone in his office. Or at least his shanty.

Helen came into the world on Wednesday, September 24 of 1913, right there in the house in Two Locks. It's doubtful there was a doctor involved and likely nothing for the pain. Annie was 45. Helen was her seventh, and probably what you'd call "an accident."

There's very little information about her early years. There are no old letters or diaries or postcards. There are no yearbooks. There are very few photographs. When Helen was born, her oldest sister, Devona, was already in her twenties and married to a man named Herman Moore. Devona had a daughter. They lived right nearby in a slightly more populated area called Charlton. The daughter was Thelma Moore. She was just a bit older than Helen. Helen was her aunt, but they were more like sisters, and would always be best friends.

Annie's other children were still home when she added Helen. They were Nan, Bob, the twins Esther and Earl, and young Harry. Nan was 20 and you might say she sort of adopted her new sister. There's a nice old photo of the two older sisters, Devona and Nan, in a horse-drawn carriage, about 1914. Each is holding a baby, or a little girl just beyond being a baby. Devona holds Thelma.

Nan wears glasses and a dress that covers her from neck to ankles. She's holding Helen, who has very little hair. It's an interesting picture, three sisters, two all grown up, and in their twenties, and then this baby, who's already an aunt, with her niece sitting beside her. And the niece is older than she is.

Somewhere around 1919, Helen started at the Sunnyside school. She was smart and a good student. She made the paper now and then for perfect attendance. She made good friends with a girl named Helen Seibert, who would visit her at home and sit with her at school and one day be her next-door neighbor.

By then Devona had added a second daughter named Genevieve. Thelma was a year ahead of Helen. Genevieve was a year or so younger. Soon, they were an inseparable trio, swimming in the river, laughing and skating on its frozen surface, sitting on huge flat rocks at the edge of the property and having picnics, visiting the Sterlings down at Dam 5, watching the kids go by with their mules and their ropes, with their boats out on the river lagging behind.

And taking walks, too, down to Lock 46 and the store with Harry, or Nan, or all of them together, for black licorice and penny candy, for newspapers and sugar, and maybe a visit with the mules for rent.

The girls shared toys. They shared mothers and aunts and uncles and grandparents. They spent Christmas together. For a while, they were the three youngest in a big family that got together often and seemed to have plenty of fun. At some point, Helen's father bought a big, rare four-door Star Car, built by Durant in the twenties. He put curtains in the windows.

There was a piano in the house. Devona played. Someone else played violin. Helen's brother Harry played guitar.

Shirley Talhelm, the only person who still remembers the old house and the people who lived there, is Genevieve's daughter.

She says, "Most of our family could play some kind of instrument. I still have my grandmother's harmonica. She used to play those harmonicas for us, and they played those for their own children when they put them to bed at night.

"And they'd strum around on those guitars, and I remember my Uncle Harry was strumming around one night, and I guess he maybe had too many beers, and he went to swing his guitar and it went through the window."

There's a picture of Genevieve with Helen. Helen is six. She looks straight at the camera with a slightly amused expression. Genevieve's beside her in a baby bonnet. She looks scared, sort of leaning against Helen for support, and just about to burst into tears.

Shirley has a picture in her bedroom of Genevieve at 17, standing on the cliffs behind the house and looking out over the Potomac. Years later, in the days of Fortran and Cobol and feeding programs into machines on punch cards, Genevieve would be a brilliant computer programmer and software pioneer. She would even be involved in the space race. But in her later years, despite all that, she told Shirley, "Those days up there along the canal with Helen and Thelma were the happiest days of my life."

And Helen's, too.

Sid imagined that maybe Helen even got to ride on a canal boat from time to time for the fun of it. Karen Gray, who has been volunteering at the Chesapeake and Ohio Canal National Historical Park since 1977, and knows just about everything about the canal, set him straight on that idea.

One day Sid bought Karen lunch and asked if she thought Helen might have enjoyed riding the boats, to which Karen replied, "Sidney, there was nothing romantic about a canal Boat."

The canal itself wasn't all that romantic in those days, either. It was suffering. It had always suffered. War. Competition. Labor disputes. Financial strife. Constant flooding. And finally, in March of 1924, a flood so devastating it put the canal out of business. It had happened before, but this time it stayed that way, closed, ruined, abandoned.

Soon nature took over. Grass grew on the beds and banks. The bottom dried out. Scattered pools of stagnant water filled with mosquitos and foul smells. The lock gates grew stained and rusted and weather-beaten. The fish had either died a long time ago or escaped out into the river.

The *Hagerstown Morning Herald* described the canal from Cumberland toward Williamsport as "a dreary waste," and "a ghost of its once former self."

But still business went on. It just wasn't legal. Prohibition started in 1920 and outlawed the production and sale of alcoholic beverages, which led to a nationwide outbreak of creative lawbreaking. Soon enough along the canal and the mountains nearby, prohibition agents were flying in and seizing huge quantities of whiskey, grabbing countless tubs and buckets and kegs and pumps and boilers.

In a raid on a place called Frog Hollow, they came away with five fifty-gallon stills, three twenty-five-gallon stills, one twenty-gallon still, one ten-gallon still, and hundreds of gallons of whiskey.

Eventually, Helen's uncle Daniel and the other Sterlings who worked the canal moved inland to Hagerstown and Clear Spring and various different ways of life. But the Smalls stayed in their house high above it all, and Helen lived most of her young years right there on the Potomac by a canal that only moonshiners used, during the so-called Roaring Twenties.

They were good times for a lot of people. The flu had passed. The war had ended. The boys were home. The economy boomed. People did silly things and new things and great things. Stunt men walked on the wings of airplanes. A guy named Shipwreck Kelly sat on top of flag poles on skyscrapers for days on end. Women finally got to vote in national elections.

In 1927, Babe Ruth became the first man to hit 60 home runs in a season. That same year, Charles Lindberg disappeared out over the

Atlantic in a tiny plane without much power and reappeared 35 hours later on the coast of France, where 120,000 people turned out to greet him. He was 25 and the most famous person in the world.

There were big stars and new styles, jazz music and Model Ts. Louis Armstrong helped revolutionize American music. Henry Ford perfected his assembly line and mass produced over 15 million cars that sold for a couple hundred bucks each. Mickey Mouse was born and Miss America. Sound came to the movies. Radio came into every house in the country, and of course, electricity preceded that.

And young girls in their teens and twenties wore silk stockings, shorter skirts, long necklaces of cheap beads, and funny cloche hats that came down over their ears. They wore lipstick and smoked cigarettes. They drank at speakeasies in the cities. They did a lot of kissing. They did the Charleston and Lindy Hop and Turkey Trot. Which were dances.

They adopted a haircut called the bob, and although it's unlikely that Helen took part in the smoking and kissing and other aspects of flapper behavior that appalled the older folks, there's no doubt she adopted the bob. There's a great photo of her at 12, looking relaxed and confident, staring into a camera in some photographer's studio, with a beautiful bob she probably had done just for that picture.

She looks smart and pleasant and happy, with a small smile and big friendly eyes. Her bangs barely reach her forehead. Her eyebrows are neatly shaped into thin curving lines, like the famous silent screen actress, Clara Bow, known at the time as "the hottest jazz baby in films."

In another picture, when Helen is 15 or so, she still has the bob, but the bangs are a bit longer and her hair is parted on the side. She leans against a tree. There's a church window a good distance behind her, and she's wearing a shiny, stylish dress with the hem just below her knees.

Helen finished school when she was 13. She was cute and popular and quiet. She was also stuck, too young to get married, not heading to high school, and destined for a few years of domestic drudgery. She had no close neighbors and no easy way to get around. She had the river and the dead canal behind her, the narrow road in front, and across the road a big field that seemed to go on forever. There were no towns in easy walking distance. Clear Spring was a short car ride away and little more than a thin strip of nothing in the middle of fields and farms and a distant mountain covered in big green trees.

The Newkirk store at Two Locks was gone, perhaps swept into the river in the flood of 1924. Helen's mom was sick a lot. Her brother Bob was nearing 30 and reclusive and probably not much fun. There were fruits and vegetables to pick and can and store. There was cleaning and washing and cooking at a time when things were still done the old-fashioned way, scrubbing clothes on a board, hanging them on the line, pressing them one by one with a hot iron by the cookstove.

It might have been boring for a smart kid in her teens in an exciting time, with all the action in bigger places far away. Nan lived in D.C. She was married to a southerner quite a bit older than her, and Helen would go visit. She had her nice flapper hairdo and flapper clothes and flapper friends and nieces.

She went to barn dances. She went to parties with her nieces and Helen Seibert. They visited each other at home. Her older sisters took them to square dances at a big place called the Gateway Inn at Row's Park, where they could dance to the music of the popular Joe Mills and His Fiddlers.

And somewhere back there, maybe 1928, a few years after the canal closed and school ended, just about the time Helen stood for a photograph with her bob and flapper dress in a churchyard, she had some kind of date with a boy named Whitey. She was 15. They only went out once, but that was the beginning of the end of Helen's simple, happy life on the C&O Canal.

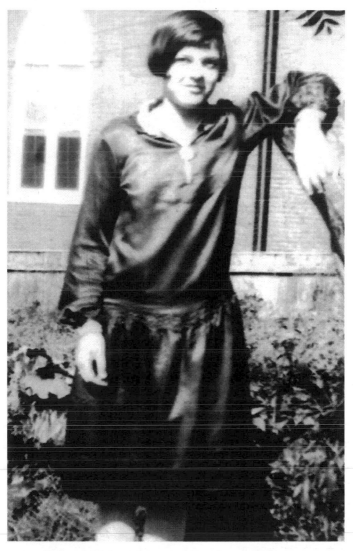

Helen at 15, just about the time she met Whitey.

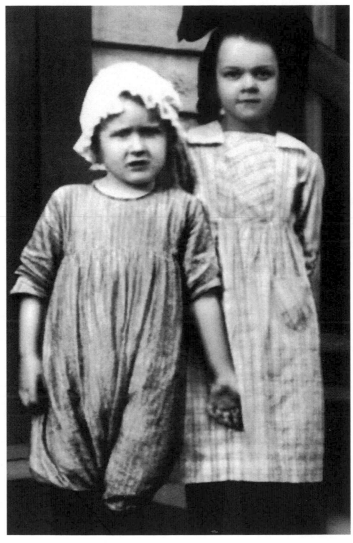

Helen on the right, with Genevieve.

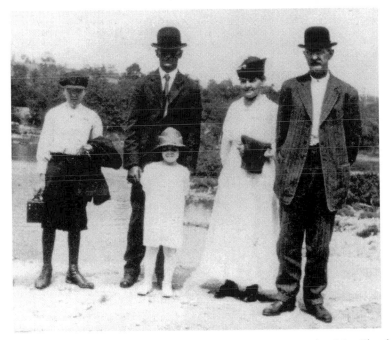

Young Harry (left), Helen, Annie, and Harry, circa 1918, with a Mr. Cloud in the back. Mr. Cloud and Helen are both wearing driving goggles.

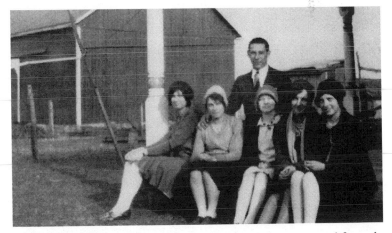

Helen's niece Thelma is first on the right. Helen Seibert is second from the left. They were Helen's two best friends. Maybe she is behind the camera.

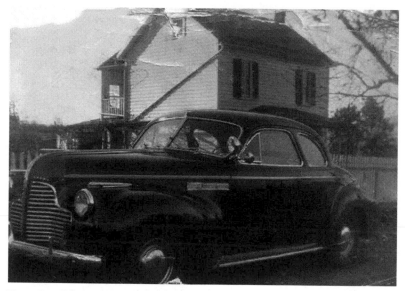

Harry Randolph Small's 1940 Buick outside the house where Helen grew up.

ALMOST ICE CREAM

I can't make ice cream, but I almost can.

SID STARLIPER

Once he got started, Sid seldom rested. You might say he was obsessed. He visited places he had never been. He spoke to people he had never met. He made new friends and learned new things. He haunted the library and the courthouse and old newspaper sites on the Internet. There was information out there, but not a lot and not that good.

The *Hagerstown Morning Herald* and other local papers printed news about the small communities outside the city under the heading of "Letters." The Charlton Letter, the Sunnyside Letter, the Shady Bower Letter, the Clear Spring Letter. The stories were mostly just snippets about the comings and goings of local people, tiny little glimpses into the past—who had a cold, who lost a cow, who fell in a hole in the dark and cracked some vertebrae, who roasted a "fine porker" that weekend. (It seems that roasting a porker was big news, and that the porkers were always "fine.")

People reported their births, deaths, dinners, report cards, birthdays, assorted mishaps, accomplishments, and ailments. A local representative from the paper would gather this information about dinners and measles and parties and porkers and send it in.

And like some archaeologist sifting through brittle things in old ruins, Sid spent hours digging through these articles for information about his mother. Every time he found something about Helen, or her family, he printed it out. He made binders full of articles. These scraps made him happy, every brief snippet, a dinner party at the house on the canal, where "all the fine delicacies of the season were served," a trip to visit her sister Nan in D.C., visits with her brother Earl's family, all the times that Helen and Thelma got together for a weekend. Every funeral. Every dance. Every surprise party.

He clipped them out, put them in his binder, emailed them to me, and tried to fit it all together and form a clear picture of his mother's life. But the clues were few, like small bits of bone scattered about, and not all that telling.

After finding the school and solving the mystery of how Helen got there to his satisfaction, Sid kept going back to the old house. It became a sort of refuge. It was calm there and pretty and quiet. He had it all to himself. He could sit on the big rocks where his mother used to sit. He could watch the Potomac and stare across it at West Virginia. He could see trees in every direction. He could imagine her sitting there as a little girl with one of her nieces or big sisters or brothers or her parents, one on each side of her, joking and watching the boats go by.

He could search around the fields behind the house and hunt for clues about her life, things she might have owned or touched or liked. There wasn't much. So far, he had found an old window frame and some daffodils he picked and gave to his sister, Betty, but he hadn't found anything spectacular. And then one day he saw a metal rod sticking out of the ground by the cellar door. He got down on his knees and dug and pulled and dug and eventually yanked out of the earth an old ice cream maker, or at least part of one, a solid metal crank on a round body.

Most likely it was Harry's.

"That was a treasure," he says.

He loaded it in the trunk. He imagined his grandfather making ice cream and sprinkling pepper over it and trying to get Helen to try it and how she would laugh and turn up her nose.

He imagined Harry teaching her to work the crank. He decided to fix it.

"I bought the pieces. It took me six months. It's almost complete, but it's very rare. A company called GEM made it, and getting parts is almost impossible. I've put a handle on it. It turns. It cranks. I can't make ice cream, but I almost can."

One day at Betty's, they studied an old picture of Helen's parents standing in front of the house. There were no trees in the yard. There was a white picket fence and a grape arbor. The grape arbor went all the way around the house.

Later, back at the old house, he noticed some interesting timber strewn around the grounds. Each was a board about eight feet long with several round one-inch holes drilled through it. Eventually, he figured out that they were crossbeams from the 5,500 some chestnut poles that once carried voices along the canal on wire that hung and flapped in the wind. Somehow Sid's grandfather had collected a great number of these and used them to build his giant grape arbor. And that gave Sid an idea.

That Mother's Day, Sid put it all together in his mind. He would throw a birthday party for Helen in September. It would be her 103rd. He found an artist at the Antietam Art Gallery in Sharpsburg, Maryland, who agreed to have a painting of Helen ready for the party in September, and he convinced a local architect, who was also a talented artist, to do a painting of the house as it would have looked when Helen was young. He gave him a copy of the old photograph to work with.

The architect needed more information, so Sid took Betty back to the house one more time, the last as it would turn out. He had his tape measure and framing square so he could get the pitch of the roof and the dimensions of the house for the artist.

He says, "And here I am, bent over, down measuring the pieces, and Betty taps me on the shoulder and says, 'Sid, you better look up.' I look up and the deputy sheriff is out front. I'd already put one piece of old wood in the trunk, and Betty had closed the trunk, and here he comes.

"I stood up, and he said, 'Can I help you folks?' And I said, 'No, we're just here visiting our old home place.' I explained about the artist and how I was taking pictures and measurements. He didn't seem too upset, and I continued my work."

A minute or so later, Betty was about 30 feet from Sid, standing by his car, when the sheriff asked if she would mind popping the trunk. It didn't seem she had much choice in the matter, so she opened the trunk.

It's hard to say what the officer expected to find, but the trunk was empty, except for a single piece of rotting board.

"Well," he said, "The park rangers are on their way. Why don't you two take off, and I'll take care of the rest?"

They didn't know what "the rest" was, or why the park rangers were on their way, but they didn't ask, and as they made haste in Sid's car, Betty took a deep breath, and said, "Sid, don't you ever dare ask me to go back to that house again."

So, Betty was out, but Sid was just getting started. He had a window frame. He had a broken ice cream maker. He had an old board. And soon he learned that his granddaughter, Sophie, played soccer with the park ranger's daughter and that the park ranger went to church with Sonny. Eventually, Sonny convinced the ranger to meet Sid at the house and let him have as many old telephone posts as he wanted. The park ranger also mentioned that the place was scheduled to be demolished soon but didn't say when.

They met at the house, and while the ranger stood guard, Sid and Sonny, along with Sid's daughter Holly and granddaughter Sophie, gathered up all the old pieces of grape arbor they could find.

When they finished, they asked the ranger one more favor.

Sid says, "There's a bunch of flat rocks around the house that must have come from down along the canal. Sonny asked for one, and the ranger turned him down. The wood was of no value, but for some reason the rocks were. And I thought, 'Man, you guys go to church together, and he can't even give you a rock?'"

The ranger did go back to the house and take off the electric box that Harry's son Earl had installed many years ago. He handed it to Sonny as a consolation prize.

THE SWEET SHRUB

In April of 2016, just over a year from the breakfast at Bob Evans and his first visit to the house, Sid returned one more time. The government hadn't demolished it yet, and he hoped they never would. But nature kept at it.

"It was overgrown," Sid says. "It was very thick, very heavy, and as I was walking around, I noticed a bush that had a lot of pretty red flowers about eight feet off the cellar door on the left side of the house, and I thought, 'My golly, they're really pretty.'"

A few weeks later over the phone, Shirley mentioned that on the side of the house, there was something called a sweet shrub. She said it had to be at least 100 years old and that she could still smell it whenever she thought about it. She told him Helen and her sisters used to pull flowers off the shrub and mash the bits up into their hankies and that was their perfume at school.

As soon as Sid realized Shirley was talking about the bush with the pretty flowers, he hurried back to the house. The shrub was gone.

"I looked everywhere. I thought, 'Oh my golly, all the flowers are gone, and I can't find it.' Well, I was down in the dumps, but at the last minute I just happened to look up, and about ten feet in the air, there was one flower.

"I had a hammer with me from my working days, with a claw on it to pull nails. So, I dug up a piece of the shrub and put it in my car. It was about eight or ten feet long. I felt I was entitled to a piece of that shrub, so I put it in through the window and out through the back, and away I went."

Fortunately, the park ranger who wouldn't give him a rock didn't see him driving up the road with a giant bush sticking out his window. Sid planted the shrub, but he was a bit perplexed by its behavior.

"Now what it does, once they mature and start to grow, they'll send out what they call a 'sucker,' a root that grows horizontally out from the main plant, and then another one will come up. Anyhow, I was afraid the first one I had was going to die, so I would go back, and I would dig up roots and take them home. But they wouldn't grow."

Sid spent much of that summer at the house on the canal, digging up roots and putting them in little plastic bags and taking them home, where he did various experiments with cuttings and root hormone and special soil. But just like he couldn't quite build an ice cream maker from an old crank, he couldn't quite grow a sweet shrub from an old one.

"That whole summer, all I was doing was taking pictures and digging up sweet shrub plants. It was quite an experience. I just loved every minute of it."

HAPPY BIRTHDAY, HELEN

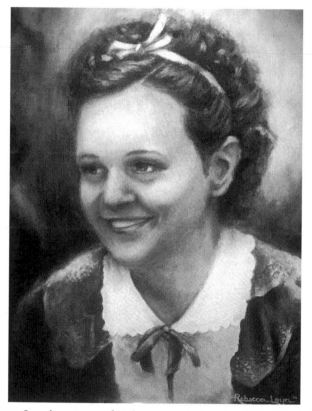

Rebecca Loya's portrait of Helen, presented on her 103rd Birthday.

They buried Helen in 1952. In May of 2016, Sid went out into his back yard in Frederick and started digging. He was going to build a grape arbor. He was going to use the old telephone posts from the grape arbor around Helen's house on the canal, and he was going to throw a party for his mother.

He got the whole family involved, brothers, sisters, daughters, granddaughters, boyfriends. They dug out the grass and the ground to lay the brick pavers that would make the arbor floor. It was hard work. It was summer. And as he dug and put down bricks and carried wood in the heat and hammered it up, Sid noticed something unusual. He went to his doctor for a checkup.

"I told her no matter how hard I work on the grape arbor, digging dirt, laying brick, I never get tired. I can do that all day, and I don't want to take a nap. I don't want to take a break. And she said, 'The reason is written all over your face. It's coming from your heart.' And then I got it. It was a work of passion. The strength came from my heart.

"And she listened to me. I felt so good leaving her office that day. And because of that passion, I was constantly looking for someone to tell my story, and that whole summer, it didn't matter whether I went to the post office, the grocery store, the gas station, I would talk about my mother and this birthday party, and people would listen. Complete strangers. It was wonderful."

Soon the arbor was up, 405 red pavers Sid bought from a brick place in Frederick for $205, resting on a bed of sand and gravel, with $185 worth of sturdy modern wood from Home Depot on the sides. And up top, the old telephone pieces from the Small's arbor holding it all together. He moved the sweet shrub right beside it. He hung a swing in Helen's honor, because when she was young and her father was a man in his fifties, he hung one in his arbor for her.

They set up cookers and chairs and pictures, and on September 25, 2016, in Frederick, Maryland, Sid threw a party in his back yard celebrating his mother's life and her 103rd birthday. She had been dead nearly 65 years. Sid hadn't seen her in 67. Her sons were all alive. So were Beverly and Betty. It was a hot day, overcast and uncomfortable. But it was a birthday party, maybe the first in Helen's honor since she turned 17.

About 50 people showed up. Sid made a short speech but didn't have a lot of good information to work with and wasn't satisfied with it. Afterwards they ate. They drank water and soda and shared stories and looked at pictures.

Then came the unveiling of the paintings. There were three, each covered with a piece of fabric Sid bought for the occasion, two green, one orange. Sid's daughters, Beth and Holly, unveiled the first two. First was the beautiful painting of the old home on the canal. Then was the painting of Helen. And finally, Sid called Mike McKee up.

Mike was the guy who told Sid how to find the Sunnyside school. Mike was in his late sixties and had no idea why Sid called him up there. He was very friendly and all smiles, but when he pulled back the cover to expose the last painting, a beam of sunlight broke through the clouds and hit directly on the canvas.

On the canvas was a painting of Patsy Starliper, Helen's last child, the one born silently in the middle of the night, the only one of Helen's children who wasn't there that day.

Patsy was dead.

She'd been dead ten years. But in the painting, she was healthy and young and smiling, and when that beam of sunlight hit straight on Patsy's eyes, Mike fell completely apart.

PEACHIE

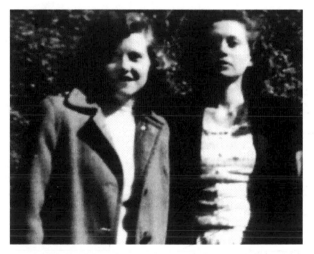

Mary Haines (Peachie), whose mother loved Helen's chicken, with Jean Charles, who cut Helen's hair.

Oh, she was sweet. She was a beautiful woman with teeth like pearls. When my aunt Helen talked, her voice sounded like music. Her demeanor was very soft and very quiet and very happy. She was always smiling. No matter what she was going through, she never complained. Even when she was in her first stages of being sick. And whatever she thought about Whitey, she would never say anything bad about him.

SHIRLEY TALHELM

75

Summer 1939

So far, Sid had only spoken with one person who knew his mother well. That was his cousin Shirley, who was nearing 16 when Helen went away. Then one day Sid's sister Beverly met a lady at the hairdressers who knew Helen. The lady lived in an old house about half a mile from where Sid grew up.

Unfortunately, the lady was now in the Meritus Medical Center in Hagerstown. She was nearing 90 and had fallen recently and broken something.

Sid headed straight to the hospital. When he got there, he realized he didn't know her last name. All he had was Mary, and there were three Marys in the hospital. Somehow, he got the room numbers of all the Marys. He was going to visit every Mary if he had to. But he got lucky. He walked into a room where a Mary was sleeping and woke her right up.

"Hi," he said, "Sorry to wake you up. Are you Mary?"

She said, "Yes, and who are you?"

"I'm Beverly Starliper's brother, Sid."

"Oh yes, I've heard about you. And yes, I know what you're going to ask me. And yes, I knew your mother."

Her name was Mary Haines. People called her "Peachie." She prefers Mary, but we'll use Peachie, since it's easier to remember.

In the summer of 1939, when Peachie was 11, Whitey and Helen ran a small restaurant, and her mother sent her over there to get chicken for lunch. Apparently, Peachie's mother considered the place more of a bar than a restaurant.

She says, "My mother wouldn't go into a bar. She wouldn't even go close to a bar. She would have called it a 'beer joint.' That's what we called them. Beer joints.

"Sidney, your mother made the best fried chicken ever. I guess it was floured and fried in lard. It was two pieces of chicken on a buttered hamburger roll.

"There was an alley there. I'd go through there and up the alley and there was a stream. Now, I don't know if there was a log over it. I went barefoot a lot, so I may have just waded through it. Then I'd go up in the back and up a couple of steps, and your mother would be frying chicken in there. There was a screen door. I just opened the door, because it was the summer and it would be very hot, and I'm sure she was extremely hot in there.

"And she'd have a white apron on, and it would be greasy, of course, and she would get me the chicken. I did that all summer. It was a quarter for the two pieces of chicken, and she was always so nice to me, so nice and so sweet. That's probably one of the reasons I remember her, because she was really nice."

Helen was nice, even when she was pregnant, like she was that summer, 25 years old and making chicken for a little girl in a sweltering kitchen with two babies already and another growing under her greasy apron.

Peachie liked Helen's company. She lingered. Helen made her feel wanted. Made her laugh.

"Not everybody in town was nice to me," Peachie says. "I was spoiled. I had everything. I had a dad. I had a grandmother, and people thought my dad bought me everything. I had a bike. I had skates. I had skis.

"Some of the mothers of my friends could hardly feed their families because it was the Depression, and I could imagine they would have been very resentful of me. If you couldn't feed your family and you saw a kid who has everything, you would be resentful, but your mom was always nice to me."

THE BLADES OF CEILING FANS

In the summer of 2017, Sid finally showed up in Sykesville. To the people of Washington County, Sykesville and Springfield pretty much meant the same thing. For some reason, most of them called the hospital Sykesville and imagined it as some sort of hell on earth where you went and never came back.

Today, Sykesville's a small town with just under 4,000 people, which actually makes it quite large compared with Clear Spring's 350 or so. It's nice, quiet, clean, and modern with lots of parks and grass. It's pretty and well-maintained, with nice children and a small Main Street that's been revitalized in recent times.

It's filled with big, new houses built by builders with set floorplans and the like on farmland in the nineties, but also with old houses of every sort and style imaginable.

There's an old train station as you cross the short bridge over the Patapsco from Howard County into Carroll and Sykesville. It's a restaurant now. There's a big old stone store across from the restaurant and built in 1866. It's a distillery now. There's an old Catholic church from 1868 up a hill behind it. It's still a church, but seldom used.

There's a crumbling blue caboose rusting on an abandoned train line near the train station. There's a gothic mansion on a hill looming over it all, totally out of place, like something from an old horror film.

And of course, there's Main Street, only two blocks long, with its bars and ice cream shops, a nice bookstore, a few specialty shops of various sorts, and big old buildings built in the early twentieth century for a man with pince-nez glasses and a nice moustache named Wade H. D. Warfield.

Everything seems sort of fresh and modern, newly painted and pretty, but back in 1950, Sykesville was a dump, slowly emerging from the Depression and the war, just an old B&O rail stop in a sea of farmland on the south branch of the Patapsco River.

The train station wasn't a restaurant then. It was a rundown 66-year-old building where freight trains pulled in and dropped coal and lumber and farm supplies. For a long while, passenger trains stopped there, too, but in 1949, the railroad decided passenger service wasn't worth it anymore.

There was a stream then, running down behind and beneath the buildings on Main Street, like the stream running through Clear Spring. The toilet in the local hardware store opened directly into the stream. So did the bathroom of the big feed store by the railroad. So did other bathrooms from other businesses and homes. People dumped their dirty dishwater out back windows into the stream. Dirty water of every sort, from dishes and toilets and laundry tubs, emptied into the stream, and flowed down to the Patapsco.

Some summers when not enough rain fell, the stream dried up and the fire department came out with their hoses and flushed the stink and refuse out of the dry stream beneath the town and out into the river.

But when people in Clear Spring said "Sykesville" back then, they didn't mean this little town with its brick station and rundown Main Street. Sykesville was the name they used for the hospital right outside town, a big, beautiful place on acres of grass and filled with old buildings designed by some of the best architects of early 20th century Baltimore.

By 1950, it had expanded to 1,500 acres and become basically a city unto itself. Dr. Ellis Margolin, who arrived at Springfield in the late thirties, described the area leading to the hospital as "just plain ordinary wilderness with a hospital in the middle of it."

But on the grounds of that hospital there were trees and fields and big old beautiful buildings. By the time Helen came in 1950, there were thousands of patients.

And now came Sid more than 65 years beyond that, with no idea what he was going to find. He drove in off Route 32, around a traffic circle and into nothing but grass and buildings. There were windows out in upper floors and doors nailed shut and porch roofs falling or propped up with wood. There were rusted fire escapes and hanging drain gutters.

He was on the grounds of what had originally been the women's wards. It was known as the Warfield Complex now and had actually been annexed into the town of Sykesville in the late 1990s. Each building was identified by a letter. Three had been renovated and put into use in recent years, but the rest were abandoned, with those warnings about asbestos on their doors and the occasional faded fall-out shelter sign with its orange triangles in a circle of black.

There were huge trees, but not all that many. There was one main street through the complex, and several side streets going this way and that. It was intimidating, and Sid wasn't quite sure where to go, and where he was allowed, and he cut that first visit short.

He went home and studied the hospital records some more. He decided Helen had been in the E building. And so, he went back to get a look at the E building. His main objective was to get a better copy of his mother's medical records. He had no idea how to do that, but he also wanted to walk around, and maybe even get inside where Helen once lived.

The smallest of the three restored buildings was the H building, originally built to house mentally ill women with tuberculosis. It was the Carroll Dance Studio now, where little girls came to learn ballet on beautifully restored hardwood floors. Sid drove in behind a car that was headed for the studio. He parked near a big blue water tower and the G building, another nicely renovated building that had once been a dormitory for women but housed a small high-tech company now.

The E building was down a hill a bit from the dance studio. It had also been a home for the female insane not that long ago, but now it was empty, old, unrenovated, and crumbling a bit, with lots of windows surrounded by peeling white paint.

Just as he approached the E building, a white Chevy pickup stopped nearby. There were two women inside smoking cigarettes, and Sid introduced himself. He doesn't remember what he was wearing, but it obviously impressed one of the women, because the first thing she said was, "Are you here to buy this?"

Sid said, "Buy what?"

"The hospital. Are you here to buy the hospital?"

He laughed. He told her he couldn't afford the hospital, and what would he do with a mostly abandoned mental institution anyway?

Then, while they blew smoke out the windows, he told them about Helen and how he would love to get inside some of the buildings. The women told him that was likely impossible, at least in a legal sense, but suggested he visit the Town House in Sykesville and see what they could tell him. They gave him directions and off he went.

The Town House they sent him to isn't really a townhouse by today's definition. It's a large old historic home that somehow became the seat of the town's government and serves as a sort of small city hall. It even served as the town's police station back in the seventies and eighties. The police didn't have a jail, so they handcuffed prisoners to radiators before they could transfer them to the county seat in Westminster, or wherever else they might be heading.

But the town's a modern place now, well-managed, with sufficient funds and a nice new police station with an actual jail inside. The Town House has been nicely restored, and Sid walked straight in. In the first room he saw, there was a meeting going on. He decided not to interrupt the meeting.

Instead he went left down a hallway lined with black and white photos of old mayors and members of town council and arrived at the front desk. He introduced himself to the nice woman in her twenties who worked there and told her about Helen.

Her name was Kerry. She sat at a desk beside a beautiful stairway built when the house was young, sometime before the Civil War. She assured Sid that no one would let him into the E building, or any other building over there. She suggested, though, that he try the Gate House Museum to see what they could tell him, "they" being me and my wife, Andrea, the two curators.

Eventually, we met, and after our second or third meeting, when I realized how much it meant to him, I told Sid I could probably get him into the E building if he didn't mind a little asbestos.

Jonathan Herman was mayor of Sykesville from 1995 to 2009. He led the effort to save Warfield and make it part of the town. It was a complicated process involving the state, the town, the county, and thousands of hours of meetings and negotiations.

It's been 20 years now, and the project is still evolving. They're building townhouses on some of the old hospital grounds, about 140 or so, but the biggest and best of the old buildings still sit there abandoned and disintegrating, waiting for some sort of rescue.

On January 27, 2018, Jonathan met us at Warfield with a bunch of keys and his really powerful battery-operated screwdriver. First Jonathan opened the E building by unscrewing a two-by-four installed across the doorway to keep intruders out.

According to Sonny's hospital records, Helen lived in S2E. We decided that meant the south end of the E building on the second floor. The E building was about a hundred years old and had been in service up through the seventies and certainly empty since long before Sid's granddaughters were born.

So, in we went, through dark hallways, past empty rooms and offices, where people had lived, and nurses had worked. It didn't take long to find E2. There was a bathroom right beside the only door into the room. There was a roll of toilet paper partially unrolled on the floor in the hallway, and the room itself was empty and probably had been 50 years or so. It was small and charmless. It had no windows and couldn't have fit many beds.

But that didn't seem to faze Sid. He walked around with a big smile. He stared at the walls. He imagined the beds. He imagined Helen lying in one.

He looked into the bathroom. There were sinks from another era in there and dry toilets filled with rust and plaster and the tossed ends of cigarettes. There were mirrors behind the sinks. There was no running water.

Sid looked into a mirror he thought Helen might have looked into. He shook his head a lot and said, "awesome," and "wow," and "this is unbelievable."

After that we went outside and took the short walk to the huge dining hall and auditorium building where women ate by the hundreds for years and years. It was vast and empty with ceiling fans way up high with their blades bent and drooping, like wilted flowers.

Downstairs beneath the dining hall was a huge auditorium. At the top of the stairway above the black railing that led us down to the auditorium, someone had broken in and painted on the wall in black, "Down to Hell I Go."

The auditorium was empty. There were no chairs. There was a stage at the end where, years ago, old films flashed across a screen and patients sat in rows of folding chairs. Countless nurses received their diplomas on that stage. Hundreds of boys and girls graduated from Sykesville High and walked across that stage, while their parents watched.

Patients danced together in there. Patients gave fashion shows for other patients. There was a big old speaker on the stage, beat up and black and probably from the sixties. There was a snare drum and a rope to pull the curtain open, but the curtain was just a few dirty shreds up too high to reach.

We wandered through vacant hallways and rooms. Every so often we would come across an old rag or piece of dirty clothes, a comb, a Band-Aid, a wig, piles of paper strewn about, broken chairs, busted speakers and light fixtures, and all the window ledges covered with chipped, cracked, and peeling paint, dead bugs and dirt and dust. We found an entire closet of old clothes worn by actors long ago.

We found a beautiful old black piano, a grand, with one leg out, down on its left front corner. The keys were chipped and broken and discolored, like a set of bad teeth. But the piano seemed more like a crashed warplane face down on a beach somewhere than a neglected mouth.

We found a small room at the back of the auditorium with an old film projector just sitting in there, a big piece of heavy technology that probably hadn't shown a film since Nixon was President and was probably made and carried in there long before that.

It was fun. It was fascinating. It was sad and nice. And a great day for Sid. He had walked through the buildings and spent time in the room where his mother lived her last days.

Except, that wasn't really the case. A few weeks later, I learned that Helen had never actually lived in the E building and had never set foot in the dining hall with its wilting ceiling fans or the old auditorium, with its crashed piano and ancient film projector. We had it all wrong.

THE RUINS AND THE ROCKS

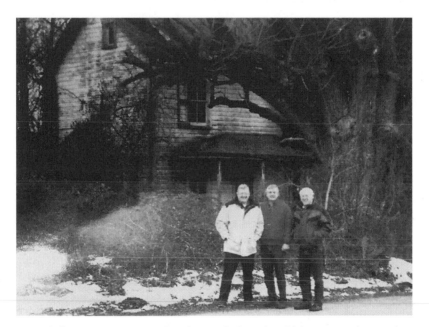

From left, Sonny, Dave, and Bob pose before the old house on the canal in 2002. By the time Sid and I visited, it had mostly collapsed.

Eventually, Sid and I agreed that I would write this book. At first, I thought there might not be enough story. Then I thought there might be too much story. At some point I realized I wasn't sure what I'd gotten myself into. I just knew that over the course of time, the amount of which was a key variable, I would figure it out. And that's how I found myself on Interstate 70 heading west toward Clear Spring for the first time.

It's easy to get to Clear Spring from Sykesville, even for someone like me, who isn't good at that sort of thing. I just got on 70 and drove about an hour, until I saw a giant pole sticking up out of the hills to my right with a flag on it and a big M flapping in the breeze. The Clear Spring McDonald's. And that's where I met Sid the first time we visited the old house on the canal.

It was dark and misty that afternoon, and Sid drove us to a small lot right by Dam 5, where we watched the river spill over the falls and crash down into white foam. The dam was beautiful and just beyond it was the old lockhouse where Harry Small's uncle had lived and tried to keep an injured boat captain alive. We didn't know that story yet, or that someone from Sid's family had actually lived there for many years.

Across the river in West Virginia was an old hydroelectric plant that started life as a mill. We didn't know that Sid's uncle Earl, Helen's brother, had worked over there, or that Sid's family had once had a strong presence all along this stretch of canal.

The clouds spit on us. We headed away from the dam, up the concrete towpath along the cliff toward Two Locks, the river on our left and a wall of hard rock going straight up on our right. Our destination was the point in the cliff, halfway between Dam 5 and Lock 45, where if we could climb straight up, we would arrive at the back yard of the old house where Helen, Thelma, and Genevieve played together all those years ago. But about ten minutes from the dam and our car, the rain cut loose. There was no point in running, so we turned around and walked back to the car.

For some reason, Sid had two perfectly clean white hand towels in his car. We dried our hair and faces and sat there dripping, while water splashed and rain poured and the Potomac spilled over the dam.

We drove away on Dam 5 Road and came to an extremely narrow point in the road. Sid pulled over by what looked like some scrubby woods on the edge of nothing. I could barely see through the rain and wipers and blurry windows. He pointed out a structure of sorts in the dark dripping brush and trees. It looked small and brown.

It was the house on its sopping perch. I tried snapping pictures, but the rain kept coming, the windows kept smearing, and we decided to head back to McDonald's. By the time we got there the sun was out, and we stood in the parking lot with dry faces and soaked underwear, and Sid took out Bernie's bat and Harry's ice cream maker and let me look.

The ice cream maker was a solid thing patented in 1894, while Frank Brown was governor of Maryland and Springfield was still a giant farm. It said GEM on it and NORTH BROS MFG CO PHILA PA USA, serial number 163.

And Bernie's old paddle felt as good in my hands as any baseball bat I'd ever held. I gave it a couple swings in the sun and wondered, "What kind of ball would I hit with this thing?"

The next time I visited was sunny and windy, 65 degrees and beautiful, with deep, clear blue skies that really did seem to go on forever. First Sid took me to a terrific old restored mansion at the edge of town called Plum Grove, where Peachie worked and raised classic roses, and then he drove me around Clear Spring a bit, where most all the houses are old, and the telephone poles are thin and crooked.

It was near Halloween. There were skeletons and corpses, witches and vampires, and that sort of thing hanging everywhere. Fields filled with the stalks of harvested corn surrounded us. Fairview mountain stood down the hilly road in the distant west, like a giant wall of trees we could drive straight down into. There was traffic, but not much and not fast.

Most of Clear Spring is actually one street, about two miles long. The street seems to have several names, which I never did quite sort out. It started out as something called the National Road, which the federal government began in the early 1800s and finished in 1837.

The road eventually connected Wheeling on the Ohio border with Baltimore.

Congress actually authorized the funds to build the road in 1806, while Thomas Jefferson was President. It was the first highway built completely with federal funds and a bit of a technological marvel for its time, much like the canal.

Today, as it runs through Clear Spring, the road, with its drainage ditches on each side, is also Route 40, Main Street, and Cumberland Street. Just about every house on the street, and the couple short side streets we went down, was there before Sid. Most started as businesses tending to the needs of horse travelers in the years before the Civil War. Blacksmiths and barbers and butchers, the people who ran stores and took care of saddles and wagons and horses.

Part of the attraction was the spring. It's still there, shallow and narrow and cutting through yards, running under houses, and not really serving any purpose that I can fathom, but once, it provided a nice stopping point for stagecoaches and wagons and thirsty horses.

Eventually, most of the old buildings became houses and apartments and stores, and Clear Spring seems very quiet and mostly forgotten now, a mountain covered in trees in one direction, endless farmland in all the others, and barely a tree on Main Street.

Aside from the McDonald's right behind Sid's old yard, on a spot that once housed an ice cream place called Tastee Freez, very little looked new. The town's just about 200 years old and a bit ragged, with a few nice old brick buildings and pretty churches. It's isolated and beautiful, and maybe not exactly paradise, but surrounded by it.

Sid showed me the Starliper house on Main Street at the edge of town. It was white and old and small with air conditioners jammed out upstairs windows. The barn out back was gone, and you could walk from the back yard to the McDonald's in a minute or two, depending on how fast you moved your legs.

A few straggly bits of dead vine stuck to the white siding out front of the house. There were old Christmas lights over the front door waiting for Christmas to come back around. There were shutters on the windows and a big old tree out front on a little patch of grass between the sidewalk and the highway, and a phone pole beside that, and all kinds of wires connecting to the side of the house. Someone else lived in there now, and Sid had no idea who they were.

Soon we left Clear Spring and headed to the old house. There was little distance between the front of the house and the narrow road we came in on. No driveway, no sidewalk, nowhere to park a car. Sid parked on some scruffy nature.

To get to the house, we crossed about 20 feet of brush and thick yellow grass. Strands of thorn pulled and scratched our clothes. Eventually we took positions near the wreck and looked inside.

About two years had passed since Sid's emotional Easter visit, and the stairway Sid leaped onto that Sunday wasn't connected to the wall anymore. It was in the cellar now on its side, still intact. The stairway that once led up into the attic lay beside it, two stairways in the rubble, surrounded by black foundation stones, dead nature, and bits of wall and roof.

There was no picket fence anymore. Or grape arbor. Or barn. There were no tables topped with marble. There was no big heavy old furniture from long ago. According to family lore, all the furniture was stolen. In one story, someone broke into the house and blindfolded Bob while a couple others made off with the tables and chairs and bureaus. Shirley even has a name.

We walked behind the house. Sid wore a tan jacket and his black baseball cap with Chevrolet on it. He tended to get ahead of me.

The wind gusted. Trees swayed. The leaves hissed and flailed this way and that. Branches banged together and creaked. Vines with sharp thorns snatched at our pants and sleeves, like bony fingers reaching up from the earth and trying to pull us down under. The grass, tall and yellow and brown, bent flat in the wind.

We worked our way through Helen's back yard, maybe 50 or 60 feet, toward the cliff and the beautiful view of the river and trees in every direction, the towpath below us, the Potomac surging in the wind, West Virginia on the other side, Dam 5 to our left, Locks 45 and 46 to our right, each only a quarter mile away.

We stood at the edge. There was a great flat rock and another two or three beside it, probably over 200 million years old, older than the dinosaurs, still there, and perfect for sitting down and hanging our legs over the side and watching the windy water churn toward the dam.

This was Helen's perch, barely changed since the days of bobs and Prohibition. It was a long way down. And straight. Possibly a lethal drop. There would be no rolling. Just a fall and a landing.

The wind snapped our clothes. It whipped the trees. There was a presence there, maybe something trying to scare us off, away from the river and the house and the whole story of Helen. Or maybe the opposite. Maybe it was glad to see us, thrilled to have someone walking around the old yard on the cliff by the water. Not a warning, a welcome. Or maybe I imagined the whole thing.

Eventually, we found a gentle incline and worked our way down to the towpath. I looked back up where we were a few minutes ago, a wall of rock leading up to a house but, from our angle, no sign of civilization up there. But Helen's family had lived there 100 years. And now one of Helen's children had come home. If only for an hour or two. And brought a stranger. And the trees shook. The river flowed.

We walked the towpath away from Dam 5, where the Sterlings had lived, till the slackwater ended and the canal picked up again at Lock 45 and then on to Lock 46, narrow, empty, wet and pretty, with puddles and weeds and slimy rocks and stones and moss, all of it deep green and flickering in sunlight through the trees. The sun shined in the deep and beautiful blue skies above the river.

As we walked the path where the mules walked in Helen's time, a single bike rider came by in fluorescent green with a fancy helmet and a fancy bike and tight rider's shorts with high-tech padding inside. He would have looked mighty strange 150 years ago, or even 50. In fact, he looked mighty strange now, and I imagined dozens of sick and bleary-eyed Irishmen looking up from their picks and shovels in 1835, hungover and homesick and terrified of cholera, watching this day-glow green apparition pedal by in his padded pants with a special phone that tells him his speed, direction, heartbeat, precise position on the planet, or within the galaxy, and how to find the nearest Starbucks.

And then he was gone. There were just the two of us at Lock 46, standing on the ground of the old Two Locks store, the beautiful abandoned lockhouse, with its green roof and big, high, white brick walls watching over us.

I guess every lockhouse has its stories. In this one in 1913, a month before Helen was born, the six-year-old son of a new lock-keeper took the family gun off the mantel and loaded it.

Then he dropped it. The gun went off and fired a bullet through his eye and killed him.

But we didn't know that story yet, either. To us the lockhouse was just another bit of pretty scenery, like the one up by Dam 5 where "Guard Lock Dan" Sterling and his family had once lived for a quarter of a century.

It was all so beautiful. I couldn't help thinking that Helen was awfully lucky once, at least for a little while.

WEENIE ROASTS

Misses Genevieve Moore, Helen Small, Dorothy Ankeney
and Grace Ankeney entertained a large number of friends
at a weenie roast on Thursday night. The evening was
pleasantly spent in roasting weenies and playing games.

CHARLTON LETTER, JUNE 28, 1930

In October of 1929, something went wrong with the stock market. Soon the bottom dropped out. Experts say the crash didn't cause the Depression that followed, but something sure did. Millions lost their jobs. Many lost their homes. Investors lost fortunes on the market and men lined up for food on the sidewalks of New York. Some sold apples on street corners.

Over 11,000 banks failed, taking the life savings of everyday Americans with them.

The Depression spread across the world. There was runaway inflation in Germany, and at some point, while communists and anarchists and radicals of every other sort battled it out in the streets of Munich and Berlin, people started listening to a shouting demagogue, a World War I veteran from Austria with an absurd moustache and a talent for churning up resentment.

But in Washington County, the young people knew very little about Hitler and had no reason to expect that things even more terrible than the Depression were waiting out there in their future. There was still prohibition. There was still barn dancing. There was still fishing and swimming and baseball and basketball and church.

And when the weather was nice, the kids still managed to pull together big outdoor parties they called "weenie roasts," just a fire, just marshmallows and hotdogs on sticks and young happy faces glowing orange in the flames and smoke, and maybe some fiddles and banjos and old-fashioned country songs.

Helen was still in her teens and one of the leaders in the local weenie roast scene. She and Genevieve threw one on the school grounds at Charlton, not too far from Two Locks, where Genevieve and Thelma grew up. Over 80 people came. The paper ran out of room and couldn't list all the names.

When Helen turned 17 that September in 1930, they threw at least three in her honor. A huge crowd showed up for one and laughed and ate and played games and sang "Happy birthday, dear Helen."

And the Depression dragged on. President Herbert Hoover didn't do much about it. Or seem to want to. Or know how to. He thought things would sort themselves out and it was best the government stayed out of it.

In November of 1932, there was an election. Hoover got 59 electoral votes. Franklin Delano Roosevelt got the other 472.

Helen was 19 when FDR was elected. She was a Democrat. So was he. FDR would win election four times. He would still be President when she turned 32, and like millions of other Americans, she probably cried when he died in office, just short of winning the war.

In 1933, unemployment reached 25 percent. Half the kids in the country didn't have enough to eat. Homeless families gathered and set up crude shelters in dirty places they called Hoovervilles. Helen was 20 and then 21, still going to weenie roasts and dances and card parties, visiting Nan in D.C. once a month during the nicer weather.

Who knows? She might have moved to D.C. herself someday, gotten away from the abandoned canal and the small towns and fields of corn and country roads and fiddle music and lived an entirely differ-ent life. We'll never know, because in the end, she crossed paths with Whitey again and wouldn't be going anywhere until 1950.

THE CHAMP

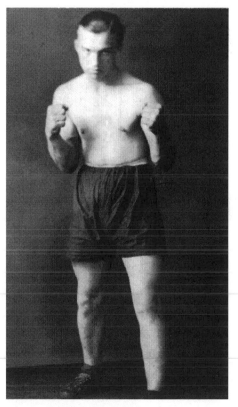

"Whitey"

He was a good-looking man, mind you, and quite the charmer. He had that black hair. And he had a lot of charisma. People liked him. But, you know, he didn't have any character, and charisma without character is lethal.

SHIRLEY TALHELM

The Starlipers were in America about 170 years by the time Helen made their acquaintance. They went straight back to the American Revolution and a man named Anthon Sterliper. Anthon was a Hessian born in Eckenheim near modern-day Frankfurt in what someday would become Germany. At the time of the Revolution, Hesse was an independent state that rented 19,000 soldiers to the British to help suppress the uprising in the American colonies. Anthon was one of them.

When Washington crossed the freezing Delaware on Christmas of 1776, he didn't surprise British soldiers, he surprised Hessians. He took over a thousand prisoners. Anthon missed that, but he ran into American forces during the Battle of Saratoga in upstate New York in early fall of 1777. The Americans took 5,895 prisoners. Half were Hessians. One was Anthon. Anthon spent four miserable years as a prisoner of the colonial army, until he escaped not long before the war ended.

Eventually he changed his name to Anthony Starliper, and in 1785, he married an American widow named Catherine Eichelberger. Anthon was 35. Catherine was 44 and had eight children. Together, they added three more. They named the last George. George was born in 1790, when Catherine must have been approaching 50.

George Starliper had a son named Henry in 1827, and Henry married a woman 16 years younger than him when he was 36. He worked as a tenant farmer and made it into the *Hagerstown Herald &*

Torch in July of 1891 due to the terrible manner of his death. "Henry Starliper Mangled by a Reaper."

Henry was 65. He was just finishing his harvest when, as the paper reported, he "was riding the saddle horse attached to a self-binding reaper when the horses took fright and ran, throwing Mr. Starliper before the rapidly moving machine. The guards retaining the knives were driven into his legs, cutting and tearing the flesh shockingly while the horses continued their pace several hundred yards."

The Smalls weren't the only ones with bad luck and terrible deaths.

Fourteen years earlier, in February of 1877, Henry's wife gave birth to a son named Samuel. He was 14 when his father was dragged across the field. Sam never went to school, but somehow learned to read and write. Eventually he met a girl named Lethean Knode, who was born on February 12, 1886.

Lethean grew up on a farm in Shady Bower, a tiny place just east of Clear Spring. She spent much of her early years with her cousin Julia Shank and other friends, sledding, going out on straw rides, visiting in Hagerstown, going to fairs and quiltings and dances and socials.

Her friends called her Lethie. She was organist for something called the Christian Endeavor Society of St. Paul's Church and played Mendelssohn's Wedding March at weddings.

Somehow early on she met Sam Starliper. There's something a bit strange about it. She knew Sam from a young age, and it seems they were always connected. On February 17 of 1898, the *Hagerstown Herald* noted that "Lethie Knode gave a birthday party to a number of her friends Saturday evening."

The article makes special note of the fact that "S. Starliper was there," which might not seem that unusual, except that this was her twelfth birthday and Sam was 21.

Whatever was going on between them, they weren't rushing things. Sam worked as a county constable, a sort of low-paid officer of the peace. He went about it with great determination. In 1906, he heard that a group of Austrians were serving liquor without a license from a seedy shack near the railroad at a place called McCoy's Ferry.

Sam decided to outsmart them. He casually walked in and requested a drink. When they served it, he requested a liquor license. When instead of a liquor license, they pulled out knives, Sam excused himself. By the time they got their guns out, he was through the door and running. They missed him 13 times.

On another memorable occasion, Sam handcuffed himself to a prisoner and went to bed. The prisoner was Harry Blair. Earlier that evening, Blair had lost a fight and gone home for his gun so he could come back and shoot the man who beat him up. When Blair couldn't find the guy, he went back home disappointed.

Then Sam showed up with a warrant, and for reasons I don't quite understand, Sam handcuffed himself to Blair, took him into a locked room, and made the man get into bed. Since they were attached at the wrist, Sam had no choice but to get in bed with him.

There was nothing remotely romantic about it. Sam got a bad night's sleep. In the morning, he took Blair to Hagerstown, where they could lock him up properly. The paper said Blair was silent and disgusted by the whole thing. And Sam wasn't all that happy, either.

In February of 1908, Sam got to name a baby. He was called to take a young woman to the Bellevue Hospital. Apparently, he traveled by horse and sled. He got the woman into his sled and headed toward the hospital, when, as the paper reported, "they were down by Charlie Barnhart's when she was taken violently ill and had to be carried to shelter in the house."

And then she had a baby. She asked Sam to name it. Sam called him "Mike."

When Sam and Lethie finally did get married in 1910 in Chambersburg, Pennsylvania, Sam was 33 and Lethie was 24. They had their first son later that year. Two years after that, in May of 1912, Sam bought the house in Clear Spring for $850.

He ran for sheriff in 1917 and won. He was 41 and an ardent Republican, with a stellar 11-year record for creative policing. One Hagerstown paper wrote that "his parents were farmers of ordinary circumstances," and that Sam spent his early years "working among the farmers in the vicinity of his home."

There's a picture with the article. Sam looks friendly and handsome in a white shirt, jacket and tie, with his hair well-combed, parted in the middle, and receding on the sides. He served two years as sheriff.

In September of 1923 he made the paper for his part in something called a threshing party. The party, at a place called Cider Spring Farm, lasted two days, and involved a lot of wheat and hard work. A man named Carbaugh, "a well-known thresherman," supplied some sort of machine that separated the wheat from its chaff, and as the paper reported, "Ex-Sheriff Samuel Starliper put the wheat to the machine to the tune of 'When the Moon Shines Down on the Farm.'"

Young Whitey Starliper and his brother, Frank, were among the 23 "men" present. Whitey was nine.

Sam's business wasn't wheat, though. He was mainly known as someone who dealt with animals. In an ad in the twenties, he reminded all those who might be interested not to forget "Starliper's Big Stock Sale" that would take place "rain or shine at STARLIPER'S BARN at Clearspring."

Up for sale were 75 head of cattle, 13 head of sheep, and 100 head of hogs. About the hogs, the ad says, "twenty-five of them will weigh from 200 to 250, 75 will weigh from 60 to 150," and one registered Duroc boar would weigh 500 pounds.

He also had some sort of business involving sheep and ran his own meat market on Main Street in Clear Spring till 1929.

His grandchildren called him "Sam," because that's how he wanted it. He seems like a good fellow, but he had his problems. In 1928, while prohibition was still in effect, he was arrested and fined $100 for driving under the influence and another $10 for driving without a registration. There was a reliable witness. Sam ran him off the road before barely missing another 20 cars and coming to an abrupt stop against the car of Murray Smith, who was minding his own business in front of the post office in Frederick.

They locked Sam in the Frederick County jail. They also locked up the $2,000 in cash and checks they found on him, about 28 grand in today's money. He was on his way home from Baltimore, where he'd made quite a killing selling cattle.

Whitey was the second son. They named him Charles. He was born in 1914, almost a year after Helen. No one knows how he came to be known as Whitey. As a teenager he worked in his father's meat market with his brother, Buck, and became an expert at slicing meat. Other than that threshing party, he didn't make the paper much, and when he did, they called him Charles.

That is until he started boxing. For some reason, when he first started in 1934, he had the short-lived nickname of "Tiny King," but by summer of 1935, he was "Whitey Starliper," and made the paper a lot in stories like this one.

"The opening bout of the evening saw Whitey Starliper of Clear Spring score one of the quickest kayoes on record when he flattened Red Miller of Boonsboro CCC camp in exactly 34 seconds. Starliper connected with a left and right and it was curtains for the 'redhead.'"

Whitey loved to fight. He loved to watch other people fight. Guy Haines, who's in his nineties now, and married to Peachie Haines, remembers, "We had several colored families in town. And one lovely lady who worked at the Overbrook hotel, she had several children, and one was a young boy who was about my age, and when he was downtown in the center of town, we hung out down there.

100

"If Bean, that was his name, was there, Whitey loved to get me and him boxing. He had the gloves and would put the gloves on us. I didn't like that at all, but Whitey loved to see us get together and box."

Mainly Whitey fought at a place called Row's Park along the Conococheague Creek not far from Clear Spring. Row rhymed with "now," not with "go," and was named after a guy named George W. Row, who bought land in the area around 1923 and turned it into a popular amusement resort with swimming and big sliding boards where three people could sit side by side and crash down into the water.

There were picnics and reunions and the square dances where Helen danced to Joe Mills and his Fiddlers, and on hot summer nights, with Joe sometimes fiddling between rounds, young men with names like Powerhouse Diehl, Kid Dawson, Flee Hasenbuler, K.O. Martin, Sambo Wilson, Wild Bill Ricketts, and Whitey Starliper climbed into a ring and tried to knock each other cold.

Whitey was a good fighter, exciting and fun to watch. He fought hard and often, sometimes every two weeks. He could stand toe to toe with another fighter, land hard punches, and take them back. He could knock a man out with either fist.

And by August of 1935, short of his 21st birthday, Whitey was the light heavyweight champion of Washington County, Maryland.

He also played soccer and managed the Clear Spring Soccer Club. He played center forward, and on March 29, 1937, in a very windy game before 2,000 people, he scored twice to lead Clear Spring to a 3-2 victory over the Williamsport Wildcats for the league championship.

On June 3 of that same year, he was appointed constable for the Clear Spring district, a position he would hold on and off over the years for very little money.

He enforced the law. He chopped up meat. He kicked balls. He knocked people down on big grassy fields and inside small rings surrounded by ropes. And somewhere along the line he took up drinking beer.

By 1933, Hitler had destroyed the democracy Germany built after the disaster of the First World War and taken complete control of the country. And Helen wasn't showing up in the paper anymore. She was 20 and seven years out of school and probably wanted to move on to the next phase in her life. In those days that meant finding a husband.

Her niece Thelma got married in 1934, and now the papers called her Mrs. Richard Brennan. At 18, her good friend Helen Seibert married a barber named Jess Hull.

Maybe Whitey seemed like a good match. Sid has a photo of him posing with the gloves on and his shirt off, wearing boxing trunks, and looking young and lean and tough. He was a champion and a small-town celebrity, well-known and popular, and not necessarily the type a quiet person like Helen might be drawn to.

But it seems he was.

No one knows where they met up again after that first date when they were 15. Or how they met in the first place, for that matter. They didn't travel in the same circles, but it was a small county. They could have met at a weenie roast or a party in someone's barn. It could have been the Clear Spring carnival, or at Row's Park, where Whitey boxed and Helen danced.

Or maybe someone introduced them. A good candidate is Helen's first cousin, Hillard Shupp, who lived nearby and worked at the Pound Brothers bakery. Hillard was about four years older than Helen. She'd known him all her life. He came to family events. He visited the home on the canal. He was there at Nan's wedding.

He lived on Main Street in Clear Spring. He was goalie on Whitey's soccer team and in the nets fighting the wind the day Whitey scored his two goals and Clear Spring won the championship.

In April of 1937, the paper reported that Helen visited Thelma. What the paper didn't mention was that when she visited her niece that day, Helen was in trouble. She still lived at home. So did Whitey.

And on the fifth of June in 1937, he rounded up Helen and his sister Leila and drove them all to the Christ Reformed Church in Hagerstown, where Whitey and Helen were married by the Reverend H. A. Fesperman. There was no money for a honeymoon. They got married in the afternoon and Helen went home and told her parents. Maybe Whitey stood there beside her.

They didn't really have any place to stay, so Harry and Annie let them in. Five months later, Helen had a son right there in that house above the river where she was born and grew up.

After Sonny was born, Whitey and Helen stayed with the Smalls. Helen's old room was available. Except for Bob, all the brothers and sisters were gone. Whitey worked as a county constable for about $45 a month. He boxed. He pulled people over for speeding. He testified in a manslaughter case. And in February of 1938, after what the papers called "an exhaustive investigation," he was indicted by a grand jury, along with another constable, for "misconduct in office."

The indictment stated that Whitey "then and there unlawfully did fail and neglect to have prosecuted persons offending against the law prohibiting gambling."

There was a bookie involved and several slot machine operators in what the paper called a "gambling racket." Eventually, the other constable resigned, but the charges against Whitey were dropped due to some strange legal irregularities.

Whitey, Helen, Sonny, Bob, Harry, and Annie all lived together in what probably wasn't a terrifically happy family. Harry enjoyed debating. He enjoyed arguing and annoying people. Whitey was what Sid calls "a red-hot Republican." Since Harry was a Democrat, there's a good chance they weren't thrilled with each other. There's also the fact that Whitey had just gotten the baby of the family pregnant.

At least Whitey got out at night. The lawyer who got him off on the charges of overlooking a gambling racket, a former Republican State's Attorney named Wolfinger, was one of Whitey's best drinking buddies. Wolfinger established a clubhouse just off the road, only a short walk from Whitey's new home. The clubhouse was an out-of-service Hagerstown trolley that once ran from Hagerstown to Williamsport. Wolfinger got hold of it somehow and hauled it out to the canal.

The trolley even made the paper now and then, for instance, when Whitey shot a fox.

"A lone gray fox got a little too close to the D.A. Wolfinger streetcar clubhouse on the canal and bit the dust before he had a chance to look around. The fox was felled by constable Charley Whitey Starliper, who with attorney Wolfinger, Paul Miller, and Clarence Repp was making a survey of the district preparatory for the opening of next week's hunting season."

Eventually somehow, the clubhouse made its way to the Hagerstown Roundhouse Museum, where it sits today, but once Whitey drank beer in there with his buddies and complained about Harry Small.

Not long after felling the fox, Whitey made the paper again, when he shot a 14-point, 225-pound buck on the west side of Sideling Hill Mountain.

A month after Whitey bagged the big deer, Helen had another baby. It was five days before Christmas in 1938. They named her Beverly. She was born in Clear Spring in Whitey's old home.

In March of 1939, Whitey and Helen took the trip out to Clear Spring to visit with the Starlipers. At some point Whitey told his father he had an idea for a business. He just needed some money to get started.

Sam gave Whitey a loan, and that April, Whitey applied for a "Class B (On Sale)" license to sell beer from the Hull Property on Main Street in Clear Spring.

Soon after, Whitey, Helen, Sonny, and the baby moved in. The Hull property was just a couple old buildings attached to each other, with Jess Hull's barbershop on the right, as you faced the buildings.

The property had advantages. For one, Jess was married to Helen Seibert, and the two Helens were probably thrilled to be next door neighbors. Plus, the Hulls probably gave them a good deal. The property included an apartment upstairs and some sort of food and drink establishment downstairs. Helen brought in some of her nice furniture from the house on the canal. She brought in her pretty china set. They cleaned and arranged and put together the most private, comfortable, and happy home they would ever have.

They were young. They loved each other. They were on their own. They had a family. They had a business. Helen's close friend lived next door. Whitey's folks were a short walk up the street. It was probably the high point of Helen's life.

Her mother came out to visit later in April. Harry dropped her off, and mother and daughter attended a funeral in the church up the street for a relative named Meta King. Then Helen treated her mother to a nice a visit with the grandchildren, and a look at her new home and her new business.

They called the place "Whitey's Grill," although Helen did all the grilling. They hung a big sign out over the sidewalk to announce their presence. It wasn't a big place, or fancy. There were wooden stools at the bar facing a big mirror. There were booths along the wall on the right when you came in. There was a dining room in back, and a bathroom.

Bathrooms were a luxury, and even though this wasn't the best of bathrooms, it had a toilet of sorts with a wooden seat over a hole that connected up with the stream. The pipes from the barbershop, the house, and the restaurant all poured into the stream.

They sold beer. They sold food. Helen cooked in the hot kitchen, where Peachie came barefoot to buy chicken sandwiches.

And Whitey got back in the ring after a year off. Boxing was hugely popular then, second only to baseball in American sports, and at the center of a great drama with powerful meaning all over the world, because of a German named Max Schmeling, a young American named Joe Louis, and Hitler.

Schmeling met Louis on June 19, 1936. Louis had won all 23 of his fights. He was known as "The Brown Bomber." He was black, widely embraced by white America, and considered invincible. Schmeling was 30, a former champ, and supposedly on the downside of his career.

But then he shocked the world and laid Louis out in the 12th round in Yankee Stadium in the Bronx. Joe couldn't get up. The Nazis were ecstatic. Hitler sent flowers to Schmeling's wife.

After the fight, Langston Hughes, the great black American writer wrote, "I walked down Seventh Avenue and saw grown men weeping like children, and women sitting in the curbs with their head in their hands. All across the country that night when the news came that Joe was knocked out, people cried."

When they met again on June 22 of 1938, Louis was 23 and champion of the world. Also, by now, Germany had swallowed up Austria in a bloodless conquest referred to as the Anschluss.

Once more they fought at Yankee stadium with millions listening by radio all over the world. It was one of the most anticipated sporting events in history.

Louis destroyed him. At one point, Schmeling let out an anguished cry they heard all over the arena. Louis hit the German over 30 times and knocked him down three in less than three minutes. The men in the German's corner tossed a towel into the ring. Schmeling spent ten days in the hospital with several broken vertebrae in his back.

Of course, back among the amateurs of Clear Spring, the fights had no international implications. Only pride was at stake. Whitey had a lot of that, and he was winning all his fights again. Then came

November in 1939 and Jennings Myers of Hagerstown, in what *The Morning Herald* called a "Real Grudge Battle."

Whitey and Myers were closely matched and had met several times. Whitey had knocked him out at least once, and on another occasion, they fought to a draw in a bout one paper called "one of the best ever staged at Row's." Myers had never beaten him.

This time they met indoors in the Armory in Hagerstown. By now, the Germans had invaded Poland. England and France had declared war on Germany, and a boxing match in Washington County, Maryland, wasn't a very big deal in a world heading toward catastrophe. Except to Starliper and Myers.

The Morning Herald talked it up in their November 7 edition.

"Interest, locally…is centered not so much around the main go between Vic Finazzo of Baltimore and Bill Bullock of Washington, but around the six-round meeting between two county boys, Whitey Starliper of Clearspring and Jennings Myers of this city."

Whitey weighed 180. Myers weighed 176. From the opening bell, the crowd stood and roared. They roared even louder, late in the first, when Myers slammed Whitey in the stomach and Whitey collapsed.

The ref counted. "One. Two. Three." Whitey just lay there. "Seven. Eight."

The bell rang. Whitey struggled to his corner with a minute to clear his head. When the bell rang again, he raised himself up and moved toward Myers. Myers attacked. He pounded his way through Whitey's defenses and crushed him to the mat again. This time the ref reached nine. And Whitey got up.

He raised his fists and watched Myers come at him. Myers hit Whitey in the stomach again. Whitey started down for the third time. But before he hit the canvas, Myers stood him straight back up with a left to the jaw, then knocked him cold with a right to the head. Whitey crumbled.

The ref counted. The crowd cheered. Myers raised his arms. And Whitey lay there, sprawled out and shirtless, no idea where he was, his days as champion over.

THE LADDER

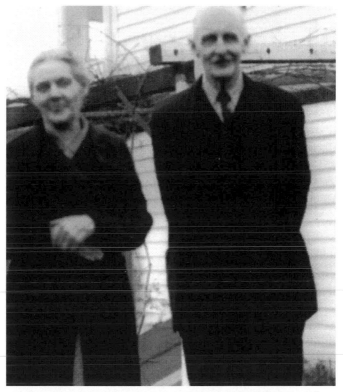

Harry and Annie in front of the old house and the grape arbor
shortly before Harry climbed the ladder to paint his barn roof.

Clear Spring, 1940, 1941

In less than a year, Whitey and Helen had to close up the grill. Despite Helen's good chicken and Whitey's charisma, the business failed. They didn't have money for rent. Whitey didn't have a job. There was a baby and a toddler, and Helen was pregnant again. They had to move. They had two choices, Two Locks on the canal, or the Starliper house up the street.

The Smalls had a nicer place and more room. But it's likely Whitey wasn't entirely welcome there or too keen on living there anyway. Plus, Annie had been seriously ill for several months and was still recovering. For whatever reason, Helen stored all her nice furniture with one of her sisters, she and Whitey dismantled the life they'd so recently set up, and they moved up the street to the Starliper house.

Sam was 75. Lethean was 66. Their son Frank was there. He was 28 and known as "Buck." Whitey's sisters were there. Everyone probably thought it would be temporary, maybe just a month or so till Whitey got things straightened out.

So, Sam and Lethean shuffled things around. Whitey and Helen got a bed and a single room upstairs, and that January of 1940, Betty Starliper was born in that bed.

By September, Helen was pregnant again. There's a picture of her from sometime around then. The picture looks innocent enough, three young women in their twenties, posing together in dresses for someone's camera, perhaps the camera of Devona's son, Robert Moore. Robert was the third of Devona's children after Thelma and Genevieve, her first son, and of course, Helen's nephew, born when she was five.

But as with so many pictures of the Starlipers and Smalls, there's a sad story behind this one. The picture was taken on the Bain farm, about half a mile from the Starliper house. Devona lived on the farm with her family.

From left to right, the picture shows Genevieve, then Helen, and then Mildred Bloyer. Mildred was engaged to marry Robert. Robert was a silk weaver at a plant in Williamsport. He drove a Plymouth Sedan, and one Saturday morning in December of 1940, coming back from Hagerstown toward home around 2 a.m., Robert decided to pass a pair of trucks on Route 40 near Shady Bower. They were transport trucks, loaded up with cars. Robert couldn't quite clear the second truck.

He was 22 when he hit the truck, and according to the *Hagerstown Morning Herald*, "Moore was crushed through the body and a hole was bored in his forehead, evidently by a piece of metal. His right hand was in his overcoat pocket when the body was removed from the automobile."

What the paper doesn't mention is that there was a ring in that pocket that Robert had bought for Mildred. He died clutching that ring in his hand.

Less than a year after attending his young grandson's funeral in Clear Spring, Helen's father decided to paint the roof of his barn.

Harry was 72. There's a picture of him just about that time, standing in front of the house with Annie. He's a head taller than her. He's tall, thin, bald, and smiling, but not much. He's wearing a necktie, well-knotted, and pulled up tight. He's in a black suit and black pants, with his hands folded behind him. His ears stick out a little funny on the sides.

Annie's smiling, too, in a black coat, her left hand folded over her right, her hair pulled behind her ears. The hair's gray and black. She looks kind of mischievous and amused and likable. It's winter. The bare branches of the grape vines stretch across the arbor behind them.

They've been together 50 years. His aunt gave him the house in 1903 and died on her 71st birthday. He's been taking good care of it ever since. He probably thinks about her from time to time. He probably wonders if he could have done something different that day when Ann Reid went for her last walk.

There was nothing he could do now except try not to dwell on it, or even think about the pain and terror in her last conscious moments, or about his grandson, either, in his smashed car, reaching into his pocket for that ring while blood spilled from the hole in his forehead.

Besides, there was plenty more to worry about now. In April of 1940, Hitler occupied Denmark and Norway, and then, beginning that May, in only six weeks, he conquered Belgium, the Netherlands, Luxembourg, and France.

Next came England. Thousands of planes bombed its cities. Parents shipped their kids to the countryside where the bombers didn't come. People crowded into subway stations. Air raid sirens screamed, the ground above them rumbled, and London burned.

Then came 1941. Hitler took Yugoslavia. He took Greece. But he couldn't get across the channel at England. So, he changed direction, and on June 22, 1941, about an hour before dawn, the German military exploded over the border into the Soviet Union with thousands of tanks and planes and millions of men.

The war was spreading. Harry knew what was coming. It seemed likely men from Clear Spring would be crossing the ocean to die killing Germans again soon. He had to wonder if Whitey would go and if Helen would come back to Two Locks with her son and daughters while he was gone.

She'd been out to visit in January and again in April. Soon Bob was born, and Harry had a new grandson named Robert. In July Helen brought the new baby, along with Sonny, Beverly, and Betty out to see Harry. It was the last time she ever spoke with her father.

It was just about one that afternoon in October of 1941, when Harry went up the ladder to paint the roof of his barn. The ladder slipped. Harry fell. His head hit the ground. His neck snapped.

Wilson Rhodes, who loved snappy cheese, was down at the river fishing, when Bob Small scrambled down the cliffs behind the house, shouting for help. People ran. An ambulance came, but it was all too late. Harry died near instantly when he banged against the earth.

They laid him out in the old house, and Helen's family gathered all together for the last time. They buried him in the Rose Hill Cemetery in Clear Spring, with the Rev. J. Wade Huffman presiding, just as he'd done a few months earlier at the funeral of Robert Moore.

Helen brought the kids out to see Annie in November, and then came December and Pearl Harbor.

HELEN'S WAR

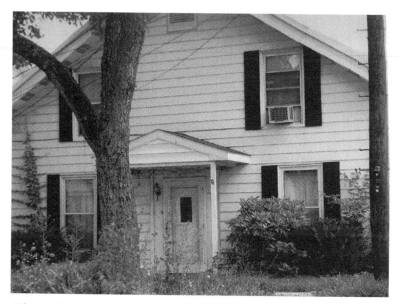

The Starliper house where Helen lived ten years and Sid grew up.

It's impossible to know what really happened to Helen. It's impossible to know what she struggled with during her last 10 years of freedom. If you could call it that. But it is possible to look at the things that happened and at least try to surmise what her life was like during the war years and beyond, when everything went bad, and Helen fought her own war within the war.

Deaths

First consider the deaths. In 1940, her nephew, only five years younger than her, a kid she grew up with, died in a violent collision. In 1941, her father fell off a ladder and broke his neck. No doubt she was still troubled by young Robert's death, when someone had to sit her down and tell her what happened to her father. It could have been Whitey. It could have been Lethean. Or Thelma. It had to be terrible.

Then she had to go see his body, dead at the house, and everyone saying, "It happened instantly." "He felt no pain." And things like that. Which may have helped a little, just like it might have helped a little at Robert's funeral.

But there he was on a sheet. It was hard not to think about what happened, hard to accept that the old house he loved had been the instrument of his demise. Hard to believe she would never hear his voice again, hear his laugh, have his help, his kindness, his crotchety humor, and his support again.

Then, not a year later, in 1942, her sister Nan's husband died. His name was Joseph Seale. He came from Mississippi. He went home and died there, and then they brought him back and buried him in the National Memorial Park Cemetery in Falls Church, Virginia. He was 58. There were three kids, and one, another of Helen's nephews, was on his way to war.

And then came Earl in 1948. It was Earl's twin Esther who set herself on fire when they were young and was saved by their mother and a bucket of water.

Earl married another twin. He liked to work. He worked at the power plant across the river at Dam 5 in West Virginia. He cut hair at night for a dime a head. He personally wired most of the houses around Two Locks and Charlton for electricity, bringing light and radio to a whole small section of the country. He brought electricity to the Small's house, too. It was Earl who installed the box the park ranger gave to Sonny Starliper all those years later.

He made small, intricately detailed houses for the dolls his daughters played with. He had a windup phonograph and a huge collection of country and western music that Helen loved. He had ten kids. They were all her nieces and nephews.

He was 49 with diabetes. One day he fell at work. A doctor gave him insulin and shouldn't have, then tried to offset the effect with sugar. Earl went into a coma, and Helen went to another family funeral.

A nephew, a father, a brother-in-law, a brother, all people she knew well and loved in nine years.

Births

And consider the births. Sonny in 1937; Beverly on December 20, 1938; Betty on January 4, 1940; Bob on June 20, 1941; Sid on March 4, 1943; Dave in September of 1947.

Five children in six years. Six children in ten. Between 1937 and 1943, she was constantly pregnant and taking care of a baby at the same time. At one point, she had five children under seven years old.

Disappointment

Consider the disappointment. They got their own place. They got a business. They had a future. They set it all up nice. They hung a big sign out front on Main Street in Clear Spring.

"Whitey's Grill."

It was going to be so nice. But it failed. They failed. Maybe because they weren't that good at managing time and money. Maybe because they were 25. Maybe because they had never done anything like this before and had no one to show them how.

And then, giving it up, moving in with her husband's family, storing all her favorite things and settling into a single room in a small house with a lot of people she barely knew who probably didn't want her there.

Things that Happened

And there were so many worries, so many scares. When she was four, Beverly, Helen's oldest daughter, went for a ride in her Uncle Homer's car and fell out. Homer was married to Whitey's sister, Leila. Beverly opened the door while the car was moving. She rolled. She screamed. She broke her collar bone on the street. She needed stitches.

Then a year after Beverly fell out of a car, Sonny got hit by one. He was six. A nice old lady named Milbrey Tosten had invited him over for lunch. He was so excited to get there, he dashed out onto Main Street, and a car from West Virginia sent him sprawling. He was knocked unconscious. He lay prone in the street. A bad concussion.

Then one night in June of 1947, Whitey came over a small hill on Route 40 and met a car from Oregon heading in the other direction. The cars hit and were wrecked. The man from Oregon broke his arm. Whitey was fine.

There were no charges. Deputy Leister Isanogle handled the case. Constable Starliper knew him well.

The War

Consider the worry, fear, and deprivation that came with the war. Helen had already lived through World War I, but probably had no memory of it. She had lived through the flu pandemic of 1918, which she probably didn't remember, either. She had enjoyed herself in the twenties and even into the thirties. She had survived the Depression. Then the Japanese bombed Pearl Harbor, and everything changed and got a lot more difficult.

Sid's cousin Shirley wasn't quite a teenager, but she describes it all well.

"To me, the Second World War is like it happened yesterday. I can remember watching the convoys go by. The soldiers would throw notes out to the girls. I can remember the women sitting on the porches every day crocheting bandages. I can remember them having dances for the soldiers up at Fort Ritchie in Cascade. I can remember down on the corner where the 5 & 10 cent store had big glass show windows, and they had pictures of every boy and girl in the service, and every day you'd go down there, and they'd have a flag—missing in action, killed, wounded, prisoner.

"I can remember the victory gardens. I can remember in Hagerstown, in front of the courthouse, there was a big old wire fence that went up way high and people took all their coffee pots, cooking pots, tea kettles, anything that was made out of aluminum, and they threw it over the top of that fence and left, and that thing would be full of aluminum. They made planes with that.

"And the rationing. You know you could only get one pair of shoes. You had rationing stamps for the kids. You had ration stamps for sugar. Everything was rationed. Butter. I remember the butter looked like lard. Well, actually, you couldn't get butter. It was margarine, and you mixed in this red powder to make it look like butter. Only the people on farms had real butter.

"Anything that was made out of nylon, well it didn't exist, because that was used for parachutes. And there were no cars manufactured. We got the first new car after the war and it came without a backseat.

"As far as tires, gasoline, that sort of thing, it just wasn't there."

The war brought intense anxiety into the houses of average Americans. Families gathered around big radios with glowing tubes inside and voices coming in from the world. They could hear Churchill and Roosevelt. They could hear about epic battles and terrible defeats, about ships exploding at sea and sailors burning in the water, about marines invading islands in the Pacific and soldiers fighting their way up the boot of Italy while cities burned all over the world.

At first, we were losing. And it was scary. The Japanese seemed frightening and fanatical. There were pictures. Japanese soldiers slicing off the heads of prisoners with swords.

And the Germans were powerful, swift, and brutal. Their army seemed unstoppable. And they were rounding up Jews.

Both were ruthless. They were "Japs." They were "Krauts." They were caricatures, but they were also truly evil.

So many people that Helen knew went off to war—her cousin Hillard Shupp, all three of Whitey's brothers, Thelma's husband James and his three brothers, a gifted young nurse named Beatrice Newkirk, who once laughed in the night at weenie roasts arranged by Helen Small. (It was her father, Harry, who made the bad decision to jump on a canal boat just in time to get washed over the falls.) Now Beatrice was a lieutenant in the US Army Nursing Corp., running the operating room on an American base in India.

Most of the women didn't go in. Instead, they took the jobs the men left behind. In Washington County, that meant making airplanes at Fairchild in Hagerstown. Before the war, Fairchild had a couple hundred workers. By 1943, they had 8,300, including several thousand women, spread across 29 converted buildings all over the city.

They ran three shifts a day, six days a week and employed most of the local workforce. They built a plant for blacks only in an old hosiery mill. They put a black foreman in charge, so a few hundred local black people could make airplanes, too. Just not in the same building as the white people.

While Beatrice Newkirk ran a combat operating room with bloody floors, while other women from Hagerstown and Clear Spring and all over the county and country, worked day and night building big heavy machines, Helen stayed home with her kids.

She washed diapers by hand. She washed Bob's. She washed Sid's. After the war, she washed Dave's. She washed clothes and dishes and children and gave them all a bath once a week beside the kitchen sink. She hung their clothes on the line. She mended shirts and combed hair and tied shoes. She looked under fingernails and into ears.

She cleaned them up and walked them to church. She walked them everywhere, in fact, and somehow kept them clean and nicely dressed.

There's a picture of the first five at a photographer's studio in 1947, three boys and two girls. Sid's probably four. He's sitting in front, wearing white shoes and white socks and shorts so short you can barely see them, his shoes perfectly tied in neat knots.

There's a sister on each side, Beverly on the left, Betty on the right, in matching dresses with white collars and white bows in perfect hair. They look like twins. They all look perfect.

The House

Consider the house where she lived. It wasn't modern in any way, or very comfortable. There was no bathroom until about 1949. There was an outhouse in the yard by the barn. There was a bedpan sitting in the corner of each bedroom.

It was hot in summer. There were no screens. They shoved the windows open, then propped them up with sticks. Things flew in.

In winter, the cold came in. It came in through the doors and windows and uninsulated walls. Sometimes the snow worked its way through the windows and front door and made small piles in the house.

The cast of characters changed often, as brothers went off to war and came back, as sisters grew up and got married, as friends and relatives came to visit and maybe stay awhile. Most of the time Helen lived there, at least 11 others lived with her.

There was no bathroom. There was a lot of drinking. Whitey drank. All his brothers drank. His father drank and even managed to get arrested for "operating an automobile while under the influence of intoxicants," when he was 68.

When Buck got back from the war, he came home and stayed. He never worked outside the house again. He didn't make any money and had none to give his mother. Whitey made a bit of money but spent a lot on drinking and didn't want to give his mother money, either.

Buck fought in the war. Whitey didn't. Buck helped around the house. Whitey didn't. One day Whitey showed up with a wife and a couple kids and kept adding more. Buck felt Whitey should contribute somehow, Whitey didn't. So, they argued. Others got drawn in. Helen heard their voices. Maybe she got drawn in, too.

Sometimes Whitey would get so mad at Buck, or one of his sisters, he would haul the entire family out to the home on the canal for a few days, where he didn't actually like it and wasn't actually welcome.

And then they would come back to Clear Spring, Whitey sullen, Helen embarrassed and smiling, pretending everything was fine.

Whitey

And consider Whitey, because everyone involved, at least on Helen's side of the family, believed that Whitey caused her problems. He was home the entire war. He registered for the draft but didn't go into the service. Most likely he was draft exempt, because of the kids.

He was home. His brothers were gone. His brother-in-law was gone. His friends were gone. All the players from his soccer team were gone, all the men he used to box. Everyone was gone.

He worked as a meat cutter for someone named Clarence Martin. He was also reinstated as constable not long after D-Day in 1944. He made the paper that August for cracking down on dog owners. The

121

owners weren't properly tagging their dogs. Dogs were running wild and chasing deer. Whitey declared he would immediately begin "enforcing the dog law to the very letter."

A week after declaring his tough-dogs policy, Whitey arrested two men for fighting at the Clear Spring carnival. He didn't box anymore. He couldn't play soccer, because there was no one left to play.

But there were still bars, and there was still beer.

Smalls

Helen's family stuck by her. She was the baby. She was the one they all watched grow up. And even during the war, with all those bombs falling and cities burning, there were good times and big laughs with her nieces and their kids.

She was especially close to Thelma. Sid recently turned up a black and white photo of them together, two country girls in their twenties, side by side against a split-rail fence, miles of farmland behind them, the wind in their dresses, their hands gently touching.

Helen and her nieces would meet on Sundays and take the kids wading in a nearby creek or up into the mountains to get strawberries.

Shirley says, "We'd have the weenie roasts, do them on sticks. Helen would come around and stay with my Aunt Thelma, and she would bring the children. So, all the family get togethers, the weenie roasts by the creek and the carnivals and the reunions and people's birthdays, we all played together, and it was just family."

Shirley's mom, Genevieve, stopped by the Starliper house often. Sometimes she brought a bag or two of clothes for Helen's kids. She never came in. They sat in the car outside the house, laughing and talking, Shirley in the back, one or two of Helen's kids crawling in there with her.

And of course, there was Nan, who was more like a mother than a sister. Nan visited often and took Helen to get her hair done by a pretty woman named Jean Charles. They would spend afternoons together. Nan was funny. They had a lot to talk about. And Nan paid for the haircut.

Helen didn't have a car, or ever learn to drive. She walked. She walked to Thelma's. She walked to her sister Devona's. Sometimes she walked all the way out to the home on the canal to see her mother. Wherever she walked, a small army of kids tagged along.

On the fifth anniversary of Harry's death, shortly after the war ended and rationing stopped and all the young people who'd gone off to war came home, Helen took the kids out to the old house and helped her mother put together a tribute to Helen's father that went into the *Hagerstown Daily Mail* on October 16, 1946.

IN MEMORY OF HUSBAND AND FATHER, HARRY S. SMALL, SR.,
WHO DIED FIVE YEARS AGO, OCTOBER 17, 1941.

Dear father, how we miss you since you crossed the great divide.
But you left with us a memory that we cherish with great pride.
It was a pleasure to be near you as we plotted side-by-side.
Now it seems so lonely father since you crossed that great divide.

In all things you could be trusted we always found you square.
And whenever a friend was needed we always found you there.
It was hard to part, dear father didn't know you had to go.
Now our meeting seems so lonely because we miss you so.
But we hope to meet you father when we are called to the other side.
Then we'll be pals forever when we cross the great divide.

Annie E. Small and children

And weeks began to pass. And months. And years. Dave was born. Earl died.

Whitey didn't make money. He didn't get them out of that single room in that small house in that small town. And Helen's hopes slipped slowly away.

123

But somehow, at least with her own family, she showed a happy face. She laughed a lot. She smiled constantly. But no one believed she was happy. Everyone believed she was trapped. They didn't like Whitey. Maybe they hated him.

Shirley says, "My grandmother [Helen's sister, Devona] used to say, 'burn these rotten pictures' of the two of them."

There are no pictures of Helen and Whitey together. Not one. So maybe someone did. But they never criticized Whitey when Helen was around.

"They'd talk among themselves, but not to her," Shirley says. "I guess they figured she had enough to worry about. She didn't get to go anywhere. If somebody didn't come to get her, then she didn't get to go. And she wouldn't leave him and go stay with her mother or sisters. With all the children, she just figured it was too much.

"First of all, her kids came first, and secondly, she's not about to inconvenience someone. She didn't want to make any trouble for anyone."

She never said a bad word about Whitey. Never complained. Never talked about her problems. And while her boys bundled together in winter, she wrapped herself in a blanket and watched them sleep. She listened to them breathe. She rocked the baby. She spoke to him softly. She kissed him and sang to him with her pretty voice. There was always a baby, Bob, Sid, Dave. And Helen was a very good mother.

And then she got sick.

Sick

Dave was born in 1947, not long after Whitey's head-on collision. There's a good chance the sickness started while Dave was an infant, if not earlier. Suddenly, it was hard to make it through the day. She was exhausted all the time.

And then came other things. Trouble finding a word. Stuttering. Trouble with her hand. Weakness in her leg. An occasional stumble.

124

Forgetting where she put things. And strange thoughts, some sort of rebellion inside her. Or was it more of a surrender? A sense that none of it mattered, a slow disengagement from the things that made life worthwhile, mainly her children. Taking care of them was hard, but it was good and necessary. It gave purpose to her life. She loved them. They were all she had.

At night Beverly slept with Betty in the bedroom next door with Sam and Lethie. And with Whitey out somewhere, Helen stayed in her room with her sons. Sometimes the rain beat on the window. Snow piled on the ledges outside. In summer, flies came in, and moths. Mosquitos buzzed her sons on hot August nights. If she turned the light on, she attracted them. If she turned it off, she couldn't see them.

And night after night, cold nights, terribly humid nights, lonely nights, she lay with her eyes open and watched the ceiling turn dark. And waited. Eventually the voices went quiet throughout the house. Lights went off. In the room beside her, the little girls lay with their grandparents. Maybe Sam or Lethean told them a bedtime story or sang them a song Helen could hear through the wall. Maybe she sang along, softly, and no one could hear except the baby in her arms.

And finally, the door opened downstairs. And it was Whitey. And she felt relief and anger and dread. She heard his feet coming up the steps. She wondered how much he drank that night. The door opened. Her heart beat too fast.

She listened while he wrestled off his clothes. He smelled like smoke. He smelled like beer and sweat and bar food. He brought a whole world she didn't know or share into the room.

She wanted to talk. She wanted to tell him all the things that happened that day. She wanted to tell him all the things she felt and feared and resented. She wanted to talk about the kids, about the future, about getting out of there somehow, about him and her, about something Leila said that made her feel bad, about how she's having trouble getting out of bed in the morning. How she can hardly wake up. And everyone notices. And says things.

Cutting comments. Dirty looks.

And she's so tired and so worried, and maybe she's sick. And there's no one to tell. Because she can't. She won't. She won't let anyone know how she suffers. But she wants support. She needs it. She needs it from him.

But Whitey doesn't want to talk right now, and she doesn't want to argue in whispers, with the boys there and the girls next door with the grandparents.

She closes her eyes. Tears squeeze out. They run down her cheeks. She whispers his name.

"Whitey."

A few feet away, Sid hears the whispering. He hears her crying. He keeps very quiet. By late summer of 1948, Helen's pregnant again.

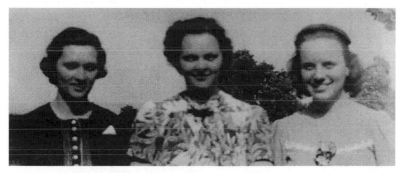

Genevieve, Helen, and Mildred Bloyer, circa 1940, shortly before Robert died clutching Mildred's ring.

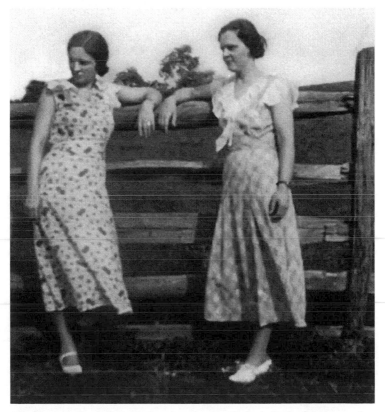

Thelma on the left with her hand over Helen's little finger on the farm near Clear Spring where Thelma's mother lived, circa 1940.

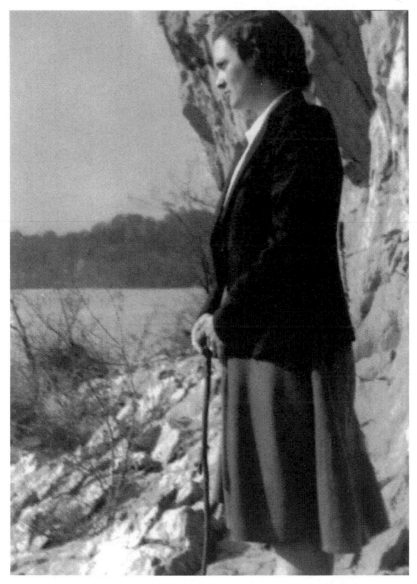

Genevieve, at 17, facing out over the Potomac on the cliffs beneath the Small's home at Two Locks.

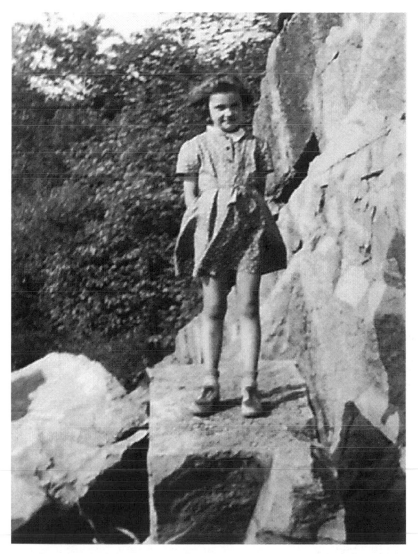

Genevieve's daughter Shirley on the same cliffs where Genevieve stood.

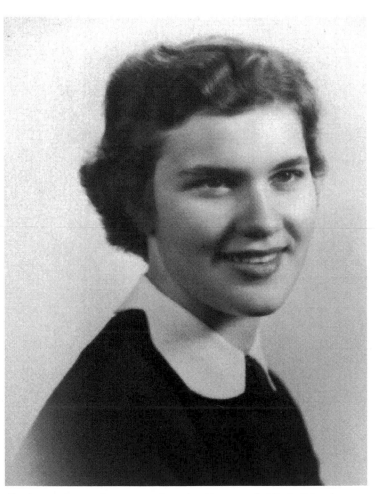

Shirley at 17, as she appeared in the Greencastle High School year-book in 1952, while Helen was in Cottage 5 at Springfield.

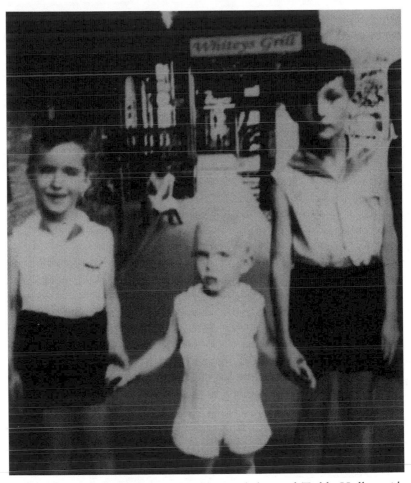

Young Sonny Starliper between Buddy Hawbaker and Teddy Hull outside the family restaurant. Teddy was the son of Helen Seibert and Jess Hull.

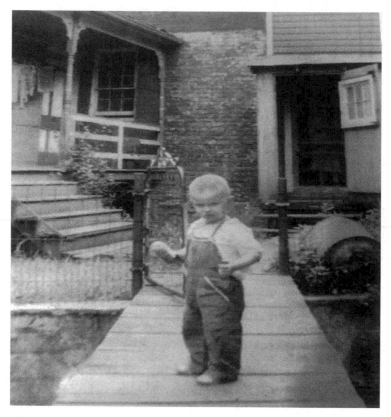

Sonny in the yard behind the restaurant, with a precarious grip on an ice cream cone. Helen watches from the door that Peachie passed through all that summer to buy chicken.

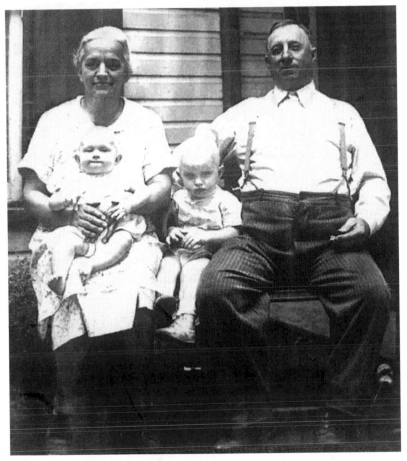

Beverly and Lethie with Sonny and Sam

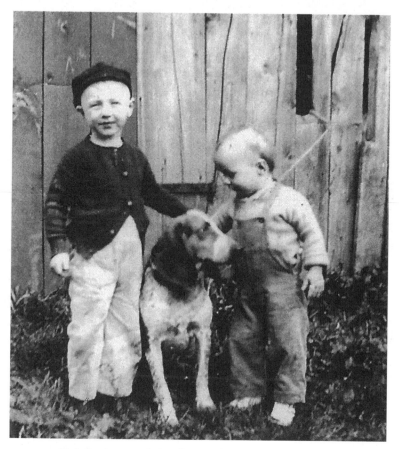

Bob Starliper with his dog, Red, and his brother, Sid.

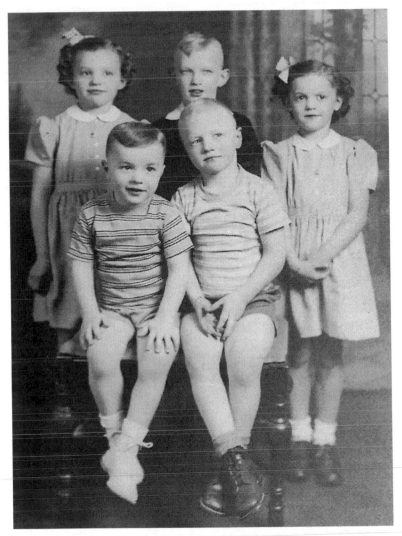

Helen's children, all immaculately groomed. Sid (left) and Bob in front.
Beverly (left), Sonny, and Betty in back.

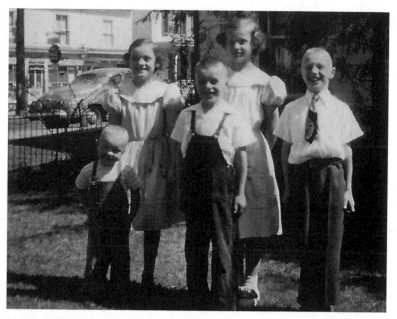

Dave (left), Betty, Sid, Beverly, Bob. Their mother is in Springfield.

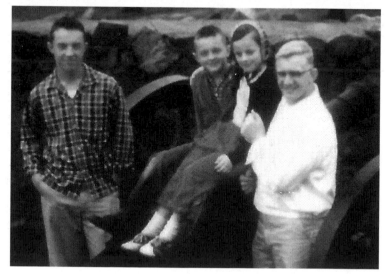

Sid, Dave, Patsy, and Sonny

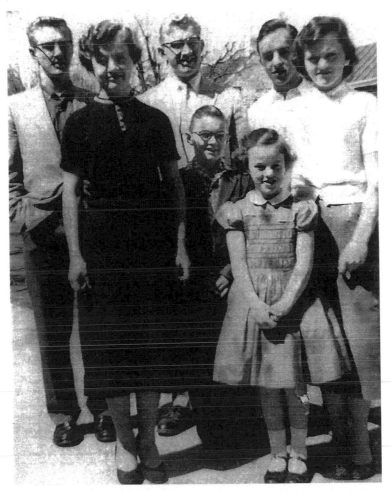

The Seven Starlipers of Clear Spring

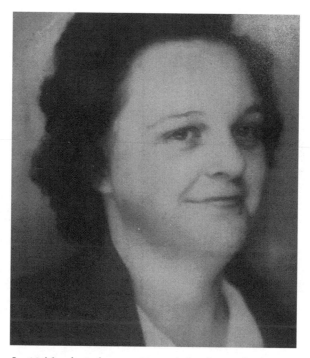

In 1946, when she was 33, and the disease had most likely just begun, Helen took her kids to the fireman's carnival in Clear Spring, where she had her picture taken in a booth for 10 cents. Is there a detectable trace of sadness in her eyes?

THE MONSTER AWAKENS

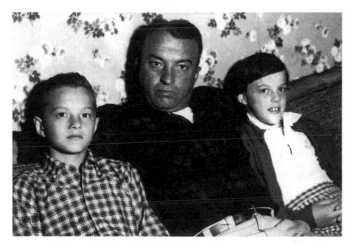

Dave, Whitey, and Patsy

*One day, your mother was going down the road,
and we were coming out from Clear Spring in the car,
and she was walking with the children, and her hair
was kind of out of place and her slip was sticking out,
which wasn't her at all, and she had a comb in her hand,
and all these little ones behind her, and that's the first
time I knew something was wrong with Aunt Helen.*

SHIRLEY TALHEM, 2018

Not long after Helen had Patsy, she began dragging her left leg. Soon, she was hardly walking. She shuffled, like someone afraid to fall down. She slurred words and couldn't always control her bladder.

After several months, she could hardly talk. Mostly just "yes" and "no."

Sid's sister Beverly is small and thin and smart with a big pleasant laugh. When Helen left, Beverly was 11 and her mother had probably been sick and slowly deteriorating for several years. Beverly has very little memory of those years.

She says, "I'm not even sure I knew what was going on when she started to get sick. None of us talked about it. I picked up on the stuttering, you know, when she couldn't talk. She couldn't walk properly."

Betty isn't much younger than Beverly, and her memories are vague, too. Mostly they remember small things. Betty remembers that Helen used Jergen's hand lotion. Beverly remembers that Helen saved quarters, or maybe half dollars, in a plate in her room to pay the doctor. She has no idea where the money came from but remembers Helen coming up to her and putting a quarter into her palm from time to time.

"That was like a bottle of pop and a pack of cheese crackers," Beverly says. "I don't know where she got the money, but every now and then she would walk up to me and hand me a quarter."

Soon, Helen could hardly get out of bed. Each day got just a little worse. Sonny would come into the room. There was a certain program on the radio, a country music show that she liked, and they would listen to that.

No one remembers if the adults downplayed what was happening or pretended nothing was going on. No one talked to them about it.

As things got worse, Helen's sister Esther offered to take the baby, but the Starlipers thought it best to keep the kids together. Eventually, Esther and Nan came and got Helen and took her to Nan's place in D.C.

Nan had always been Helen's biggest advocate. By the time Helen started school, her mother was 50 and Nan was 25. At 26, Nan still lived at home and worked as a government stenographer. At some point, she moved to Washington. In 1921, when she was 28, she married Joseph Seale at St. John's Reform Church in Clear Spring.

Now Helen was 35. Nan was 55 and going through her own terrible time. In the past few years her father had fallen from a ladder and broken his neck, her husband had died of cancer, her brother had died, her mother was sickly and living with Esther, and now her favorite sister was vanishing right before her eyes, leaving someone else behind, someone who looked like Helen, but was only partly her.

Nan brought Helen to a doctor in the city. It was summer. 1949. The world was putting itself back together. The economy was booming. Americans were having lots of babies.

Helen stayed three months in Washington. She saw the doctor. There's no record of who he was or how many times she saw him. In the end, the doctor told Nan there was nothing he could do for her sister.

He did at least name the disease. He called it "multiple sclerosis."

COMMITTED

*Today commitment to a state hospital is usually a
traumatic experience both for the patient and for his
relatives—sometimes it is even more difficult for the
relatives than for the patient, although there are
relatives who, consciously or unconsciously, look upon
it as an escape from a painful responsibility.*

HENRIETTA B. DEWITT, 1947, DIRECTOR OF
SOCIAL SERVICE, SPRINGFIELD HOSPITAL

Helen returned to Clear Spring and the family doctor with her diagnosis and not much else. The family doctor was David Brewer, a veteran of the First World War, who knew Helen and her family well.
He lived with his wife and kids in the former Hotel Potomac, a 100-
year-old hotel at Cumberland Street and North Martin in Clear
Spring. When the hotel closed in the thirties, Dr. Brewer and his family moved in.

He made good use of it. When Betty was five and had her tonsils
out, the doctor kept her overnight. There was another girl there, too,
for the same reason. The girl was 16. The girl's mother brought her
two ice cream cones. The girl wasn't feeling well enough to eat them,
so Betty ate both. Then Helen showed up with Betty's favorite doll,
and everything was all right.

Dr. Brewer took care of Beverly when she fell out the back of her
Uncle Homer's car and broke her collar bone. A year later, when

Sonny nearly threw his life away in a rush to lunch, Dr. Brewer took him in. Sonny spent two weeks in the old hotel, under the care of Dr. Brewer and his wife Edna.

He had always fixed her kids, but Dr. Brewer had no idea how to fix Helen. He had never seen anything like her symptoms. He hardly recognized her. The change was astonishing. She lay in bed and stared. He asked her questions and she didn't answer. It was painful to watch her walk. More painful to watch her struggle to speak. He recommended they take her to the Mental Hygiene Clinic in Hagerstown.

But the doctors at the clinic were baffled, too, and they recommended "Sykesville."

People had lots of exaggerated notions about Sykesville. One was that it was easy to get someone in.

Shirley says, "When I was a kid, my understanding of Sykesville was if you had problems with someone like your wife or your husband, you said, 'They're crazy. They're not all there.' If a man wanted to get rid of his wife, or whatever, you put them in a mental institution, and then you were free to do whatever you wanted, and they could never get out.

"That was the thing, growing up in the thirties and forties. If you wanted to get rid of somebody, just say they were mentally ill. You could have your wife committed. You didn't have a bunch of doctors and so forth that said 'Oh no, no, no.' And then she could never get out, and you could get divorced. That was always the understanding."

Whether that had ever been the case, it was no longer so. In 1949, there were three ways into Springfield. You could request a voluntary commitment. A court could send you. Or your family could have you committed with an official certificate of commitment from the office of the county commissioners.

To get that certificate, the family needed recommendations from two doctors with no familial connection to the patient, no relationship with Springfield Hospital, and at least five years practicing medicine in Maryland, who were willing to state that the patient should be committed. Both doctors would have to fill out an official commitment certificate provided by the state's Department of Mental Hygiene.

On July 12 of 1950, Dr. Brewer filled out the first commitment form. On the form he wrote that he had attended Jefferson Medical College and had personally examined Helen Elizabeth Starliper, age 36.

Under physical condition, he described Helen as "emaciated." He wrote, "Talks incoherently. Only answers yes or no. Walks with difficulty, short steps, drags her feet. Incontinent part of the time. Indifferent to her children."

He said that when she was five months pregnant, she "lost interest in her home and family" and was "generally confused." He wrote that she didn't "arouse anyone until after the birth" of her last child.

At the bottom, outside the boundaries of the form, Dr. Brewer wrote in ink, "This patient should be admitted to institution immediately for the safety of patient and others."

The other doctor, Ralph F. Young of Williamsport, studied at the University of Maryland. He did his form on July 17. Unlike Dr. Brewer, who filled his out by hand, Dr. Young typed his answers into the appropriate spaces, or at least close to them.

He wrote that Helen suffered from "Schizophrenia (Dementia Praecox) the catatonic type." He wrote that this was "a case of split personality arising on the basis of personality inadequacy, resulting in an inability to meet the demands of adult adjustment and characterized by progressive withdrawal with contact of persons and activities in her environment and a regression to a childhood type of feeling and acting."

He wrote of "a childish inconsistency of thought." He said that Helen would "lie in bed immobile and give no obvious response to external stimulation."

He wrote of poor judgment and lack of logical thinking. He said that she had lost interest in her surroundings and had descended into "an apathetic, dependent state of existence."

Both doctors indicated that Helen was not completely bedridden, did not hallucinate, and was not suicidal. Neither doctor mentioned multiple sclerosis. While Dr. Young offered schizophrenia of a catatonic type as the cause of Helen's behavior, Dr. Brewer offered no name for her affliction.

A week after Dr. Young signed the final doctor's certificate, Whitey took his notes from the two doctors to the county offices in Hagerstown and got his certificate to commit his wife.

ORDERED by the County Commissioners of Washington County, this 24th day of July, 1950, the statute of law of the State having been fully complied with, that Helen Elizabeth Starliper, be, and she is hereby committed to Springfield State Hospital for the Insane…

That wasn't exactly the name of the hospital anymore, but it didn't matter. The county clerk signed the form. It was official.

She was under the control of the state of Maryland. She had seven children, 11 and younger. Over 10 years had passed since they lost Whitey's Grill and their small apartment and moved in with the Starlipers.

She was finally out of there. She would never be back. She was officially insane.

THE RIDE

Sid met a woman I'll call Catherine who wanted us to understand what happened to Lethean the day she got in the car with Helen and the deputy sheriff.

Catherine says, "Even as a teenager I was aware that something was wrong with my mother. But I was never quite sure what it was."

In the middle of a conversation, her mother would just stop. Her eyes would go blank. She would stare. Her mother was Bonnie. When Bonnie reached her fifties, she got worse. By then, Catherine was married with kids and living in another state. She mostly saw Bonnie during the summer and Christmas.

Bonnie got so bad that her husband paid for a month at a facility in Hagerstown called Brook Lane, where they diagnosed her with dementia. After a month, they brought her home, and she kept getting worse. She would leave the house and get lost. Finally, her husband locked her in her room, and the family decided Bonnie needed to go somewhere.

Catherine came home for the first time in several weeks.

She says, "When I came into the house, my mother had a slip on, and she was running around jumping up on the furniture. It was terrible. And she didn't know who I was. She kept looking at me, and she said, 'I used to have a daughter named Catherine, and you look like her.' And after a while, she asked me who I was."

Catherine's brother was married to a woman named Grace. Grace called all the nursing homes she could find and anyplace else she thought might help, but no one wanted Bonnie, or if they did, the family couldn't afford it. Eventually, they realized they had no choice.

"She would have to be taken to...well we called it Sykesville," Catherine says. "But I know it's Springfield."

On the day they took Bonnie in, Grace told Catherine to bring Bonnie to the hospital. She said they would put her in an ambulance and take her to Springfield.

"So, I helped her get dressed," Catherine says. "And we took my mother down to the hospital. She was fine in the car. And when we got to the hospital, the sheriff was there. And there's a police car, and Grace said, 'I didn't want to tell you this till you got here, but she has to go with the sheriff. I didn't want them coming up to the house, but she has to go with them.'

"They put my mother in the back of the car with two prisoners, and Grace and I drove down in the back of...I can't stand this. I'm not a person that cries, but I just lost it in the car when we followed her.

"When we got down there, then of course, I was the person who had to sign the papers. And we're sitting in there at Springfield waiting for some papers, and my mother looked at me, and then she said, 'Catherine, am I at Sykesville?'

"Well this just broke me up. I lost a husband. I lost a grandchild. But I will tell you that day at Sykesville was the hardest day of my life.

"This is the first I've ever talked about it. I never even told my second husband. Just watching her sit there between those two prisoners riding down there in the sheriff's car, it was really, really bad. It's very hard for me to tell that story. I can remember it just like yesterday."

Sitting on the grass outside the Hubner Building, Catherine filled out the paperwork to turn her mother over. Then she went home.

"I would go see her with my son about every two weeks," she says. "They'd bring her out. She would be tied in the chair, because they were afraid she would wander. The restraints were around her waist, not her arms.

"She choked to death. That's how she died. That was part of the disease. Then after she died, they did an autopsy, and she had Pick's disease."

Bonnie lived three years at Springfield.

Catherine says, "Grace never told her children that their grandmother was in a mental institution, and for some reason, this is something to be ashamed of, but I don't think that way."

1950—SPRINGFIELD

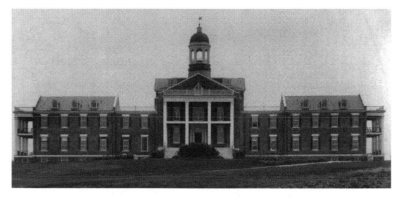

The Hubner Building. *Courtesy of the Gate House Museum.*

They were kind to Sid at Springfield. Paula Langmead, who's run the place for many years, gave him a tour. And in late August of 2018, the records office, which works out of a converted dairy barn, transferred a complete copy of Helen's hospital records from microfilm to paper and provided him a copy for a small fee.

I showed some of those records to a man in his nineties named Guy Haynie. Guy worked in the men's wards right after serving in World War II. He has what seems like a photographic memory of the past. After looking at Helen's records, he drew a map of the Hubner Building. The records say Helen lived in S2A and then E2 and eventually moved to the colony.

Guy explained that S2A and E2 were not buildings in the Women's group. They were wards in Hubner. S meant south. E meant east.

And 2 indicated the second floor. Helen had lived in two separate wards on the second floor of the Hubner building. She had never lived in the Warfield Complex.

The town of Sykesville is named for James Sykes, who came over from England with his parents when he was very young. He eventually moved into the area, started a cotton factory along the Patapsco river, brought over skilled workers from England, built houses for them, and enjoyed a brief period of success.

He also built a great hotel for railroad travelers and the many visitors from Baltimore who overran the area each year to escape the oppressive Baltimore summers. In 1868, after a massive rainfall, the river flooded and washed away the cotton mill, the hotel, and most of the town in a matter of minutes.

Sykesville rebuilt on the north side of the river. They even moved an entire church, St. Paul's, carrying it across stone by stone and putting it back together again.

Although the town is named for Sykes, Frank Brown was more important to its eventual development. Brown lived just outside today's town limits on a farm called "Brown's Inheritance." Brown's Inheritance bordered the larger Springfield estate owned by the Pattersons, which Brown eventually bought and combined with his own farm.

In 1892, Brown became the only person from Carroll County ever elected governor of Maryland. After his wife died and he failed to win a second term, he moved to Baltimore and sold most of his land in the Sykesville area, including a few hundred acres and everything on them to the state for the construction of a mental institution.

Three months after the state acquired the property in 1896, the first patients began to arrive. There's been a hospital there ever since. In 1950, when Helen arrived, Springfield was already nearing 55 years old. It was a city unto itself with 79 buildings, 4,000 patients, and a large workforce.

People from the area built their whole lives there. They worked on its farms and wards and kitchens. They worked as nurses and attendants, as doctors and accountants and clerks. They answered telephones. They cleaned wards. They fed patients. They cooked for them and cleaned up after them.

It was a self-sustaining colony of care, bordered by a small town, and surrounded by farmland. A man named David Sorflaten, who's about 90 now and lives in Rock Creek, Maryland, grew up in a home on the institution's grounds. He sent me a long, interesting letter with his recollections of the amazingly self-sufficient Springfield of the thirties and forties and the years leading up to Helen's arrival.

He says, "They supplied their own milk, chicken and eggs, pork, fruits, and vegetables, all grown on the grounds. They canned fruit and vegetables in season, kept potatoes and apples in a large root cellar.

"The leftovers from the patients' meals were collected and sent to the hog farm, where they were dumped into a large steaming caldron to sterilize and cook them, and then fed to the hogs. In late August, you could smell for miles the odor of sauerkraut being brined in the cannery.

"All this was possible only because the patients did much of the work. I remember in summer seeing the attendants with groups of women patients in the fields picking okra, peppers, tomatoes, cucumbers, and other vegetables."

In 1953, a man named William Shipley spoke to a local Rotary Club. Shipley was the chief purchasing agent for the hospital and lived nearly forty years in the house that's now the Gate House Museum. He told his audience that the hospital had its own cannery, its own machine shop, its own ice plant and laundry, its own carpenter shop, blacksmith shop, and chicken farm. It had a piggery, with 275 hogs and pigs, and its own powerplant that burned 17,000 tons of coal every year and produced the steam for cooking and all the heat and all the light.

The hospital pumped and filtered about 1,300,000 gallons of water a day. It ran its own railroad with three and a half miles of track that brought in coal from the station in Sykesville. The so-called "dinky train" crossed over Main Street on a bridge, traveled behind back yards, and across Springfield Avenue, right past Sykesville High School, then onto the grounds of Springfield and up to the powerplant.

There was a 788-acre farm. Each year, they canned 28,000 gallons of tomatoes, kraut, apple butter, apple sauce, peaches, and pears. They produced 22,000 dozen eggs and 16,000 live poultry. They washed 10,000 pounds of linen and clothing every day. They made their own clothes for the women. They made uniforms for the nurses.

There were four barbers. There were three beauty salons, where women got manicures and perms. There were fashion shows put on by the patients. There was a training school for nurses, an orchestra, a band, a choir, two gymnasiums, and an auditorium where patients watched movies six days a week.

Sorflaten, whose father, Alvin Sorflaten, was hired to set up the Springfield dairy operation, writes that "without the work of the inmates it would not have been possible to run such a large operation, milking well over a hundred cows three times a day, feeding them, pasteurizing and hauling the milk and cleaning the stalls and getting rid of all the manure, which was stored behind the barns until it could be loaded into manure spreaders for fertilizing the fields...

"You found men all over the grounds during the day. I'm sure they ate breakfast and supper at their dining rooms and had a bed check at night, but otherwise they did whatever they wanted with little or no supervision.

"There were several men who had little camps set up behind the dump where they had taken refuge in the lumber and made lean-tos, dug little caves for their possessions, and even had small gardens beside the little stream that ran there. Others wandered along the stream, and still others just hung around the barns and dairy and other outbuildings.

"The haylofts above the dairy barns was a favorite place for many of them, who kept quite elaborate storage chests, heavily locked, with their personal possessions, apparently condoned by the staff."

Most people who have lived in and around Sykesville all their lives say Springfield was the only thing that kept the town going after the Depression and the war and that the hospital was deeply embedded in the community.

Patients walked into town. When a patient escaped, a whistle went off and you could hear it miles around. Hundreds of people from the town volunteered at the hospital. Generations worked there, grandmothers and daughters and daughters of daughters. In the earlier years, many came up from the south looking for work. Helen Ferguson's grandmother came up and found work as a nurse. Then Helen's mother took a job there as a nurse. Then Helen took a job there as a nurse. Many a married couple met for the first time at Springfield.

Jeff Barnes, who graduated from Sykesville High in the seventies, walked over to Springfield and got a job that day. When he reported to his boss, he already knew her quite well. She was his mother.

There was also a staff of highly educated psychologists, psychiatrists, and doctors. Several came across the sea to escape Hitler. They spoke with German accents and had dramatic stories.

Dr. Herman Salomon walked with a limp. Rumor was he'd been tortured by the Nazis and escaped and came to Springfield. He was actually there because of his wife, Eva Rosenberg, and he had not been tortured by the Nazis.

Born in Berlin, the well-off daughter of highly cultured German Jews, Eva was adamantly opposed to war. She refused to eat when her brother Ludwig was sent to the front during the First World War.

She met Herman at the University of Freiburg, married him in 1925, and lived 13 years of what she called the life of "a lady of leisure," as a German doctor's wife. She thought Hitler was ridiculous. In 1986, she told the *Carroll County Times*, "His German was terrible. We were such intellectual snobs we didn't take him seriously."

But after a Nazi official visited with questions about their finances, she convinced Herman they had to get out of there. Soon they sailed for New York. Herman wasn't certified to practice medicine in the United States. Eva worked as a peddler in New York City. She sold stockings. She sold aprons. She made just enough to keep them from starving.

She trained as a nurse. Herman went to art school. He dabbled at becoming a sculptor. Eva paid for his schooling. She paid for her own. One day she heard of a job at a place in Maryland called Springfield and urged him to apply. He said, "no." She said she would leave him.

So, he came to Springfield. Somehow, they qualified him to practice in America. One day, he would sit among a group of doctors and hear the case of Helen Starliper.

Eva joined him 18 months after he got there. She was a nurse now. Later she would become a well-respected social worker and protégé of a woman named Henrietta DeWitt. She liked working with the mentally ill.

She told the *Times*, "I had thought they were all raving maniacs. I was surprised that I could talk to them."

Dr. Kurt Glaser escaped Europe in October of 1939 on a ship called the President Harding, which sailed into a hurricane. In an interview with Annie Boteler, whose grandfather Jack Ruby once worked at Springfield, Glaser said, "This was 1939. America was not at war, yet. The Atlantic was full of German submarines. The boat I was supposed to get on was a French boat that left New York and went back to France, but turned all the lights, signals, radio, everything off not to be caught by the German submarines. So, no one knew where it was or when it would arrive.

"I got on the President Harding instead. America being a neutral country, we had the American flag painted on the sides, painted on the back, flags on top. Then we got the notification message that a British boat was torpedoed. So, the captain of our ship made the decision to go after these people and save them, even though he knew that we were going into a hurricane. It was a right decision because we survived and saved the sailors in their lifeboats. And then of course, the hurricane almost took our ship down.

"After the storm, we had about 98 injured people on board, because the boat tilted so rapidly, people sailed down the corridors, ended up with broken backs...so one of the stewards knew I was a doctor (just out of medical school). So, he said, 'Come with me.'

"And we went, and we worked with injured crew and passengers, and there was one official ship doctor on board and four or five others who were passengers. We all worked."

Dr. Glaser's father died in Vienna. Three uncles went to Auschwitz. They were gassed and burned. His mother and brother made it to Palestine.

He had a connection at Springfield, Dr. Irene Hitchman. He knew her from his younger days in Innsbruck, Austria.

"I grew up in the Alps," he says. "She grew up in the Alps. Her father was the rabbi of Innsbruck, and I had Bar Mitzvah under him...And then, of course, came the Holocaust, and she went to Shanghai, and I went to Switzerland, and we had lost each other completely."

Though much of the upper staff were European, there were plenty of Americans. Henrietta DeWitt, a brilliant social worker, transformed the relationship between psychiatrists, psychologists, and social workers, and created several innovative programs to help move patients out of the institution and back into society. Many of the patients improved, or even fully recovered, but had nowhere to go. She would find people in the community who would actually take them in. It was a long, complicated process.

Another interesting character was an eccentric Jewish pathologist from Port Arthur, Texas, named Dr. Ellis Margolin. He was hired in 1938 to set up the hospital's pathology unit for $2,000 a year, plus a house to live in. Conditions were so primitive when Margolin arrived that he resorted to using his own microscope rather than the antiquated equipment in the rundown laboratory on the third floor of the Hubner Building. The lab was right beside the operating room and around the corner from a small supply closet, an X-ray machine, and a darkroom.

When David Sorflaten graduated from Sykesville High in 1949, he went to work in Margolin's lab. He learned basic hematology and X-ray procedures. He learned urinalysis testing. He learned to handle dead bodies.

In 1973, Dr. Margolin wrote a farewell letter to the hospital and described in detail the morgue where Sorflaten worked among the dead.

> A rusty iron table in the center is where I did the autopsies. It had no plumbing and no suction and no water. A sink along the wall was where the spigots for water were present and alongside the sink, I had to do the dissections. A tremendous refrigerator was present in the wall leading towards the elevator and two trays for bodies were present in this refrigerator. The door into this room and the windows had clear glass and anybody who wanted to could look into this room. I finally obtained some material of plastic nature that covered these windows.

Dr. Margolin was depressed by the situation and on the verge of quitting when a young man named Jack Ruby (Annie Boteler's grandfather) showed up to work as a laboratory trainee. Ruby had just graduated from Western Maryland College, in Westminster. (Today, it's McDaniel College.) Dr. Margolin gave him a book of techniques. Ruby read it, did the techniques once, and very quickly developed techniques of his own that were more efficient than those in the book.

Dr. Margolin promoted Jack Ruby from trainee to technician and raised his salary to $60 a month.

When David Sorflaten showed up, he was equally impressed by Ruby. He writes, "The head of the lab was Jack Ruby, a muscular, compact man, who could have done anything he wanted to, as he was so intelligent, but he sacrificed any chances of fame and fortune, because he wished to continue living in the community. He was multi-talented, and not only an excellent bowler, softball pitcher, and consistently ranked in the top three of Maryland's best horseshoe pitchers.

"Also, he searched for and collected Indian arrowheads from the many farm fields of the area. He had an uncanny insight as to where Indians might have camped, lived, or hunted, and he would sometimes take me along as we scoured newly plowed and planted corn-fields in the spring on various farms."

(The Gate House Museum has some of Jack Ruby's arrowheads, and his daughter, Barbara Miles, has a large collection.)

One of the doctor's primary duties was conducting autopsies, and Sorflaten was an important part of the operation.

"It was my job to go down to the morgue in the basement, take the body from the slab in the coffer, unwrap it from the paper shroud, and lay it out on the stainless-steel operating table, put out the cutting knives, reciprocating saw, and the scale, and measuring devices. I don't recall whether I sawed the opening in the skull from which to remove the brain or opened the chest cavity. After that I called Dr. Margolin that the patient was ready, and he came down to perform the autopsy. I helped measure and weigh body and intestinal parts as needed and even strip intestines for his inspection.

"After the autopsy was complete, I was left to sew up the body openings with the old baseball stitch, clean up the instruments, put everything away, re-shroud the body, and slide it back into the coffer on the slab. All this was usually about a four- or five-hour job, and by the time it was over, I was tired, bloody, and prayed no one else would die in the near future."

Between Dr. Margolin's arrival and his departure in 1973, he did 2,847 autopsies.

Aside from autopsies, Sorflaten and Margolin collaborated on something else. It was Dr. Margolin who initiated the policy of taking photographs of new patients as they arrived at Hubner. He began in 1940 with his own camera. Eventually, Sorflaten inherited the job. He developed the film and printed the pictures in the Hubner basement.

There's a good chance it was David Sorflaten who took the photograph of Helen when she arrived at Springfield. In fact, there's a good chance that David Sorflaten took the last photograph ever taken of Helen Starliper.

BURNED BY THE SUN

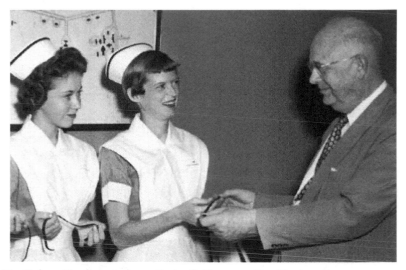

Dr. Robert Gardner and two Springfield nurses. Dr. Gardner became Springfield Superintendent in 1949, the year before Helen's arrival. Courtesy of Gate House Museum.

Springfield was a troubled place when Helen got there, slowly recovering from a blow to its reputation and morale. A recent series in the *Baltimore Sun* newspapers had exposed a Maryland mental health system that was overcrowded, underfunded, and inhumane.

Dr. George H. Preston, the Commissioner of Mental Hygiene and the man responsible for the state's five mental institutions, had actually put the paper up to it. For years, the state had ignored his increasingly urgent requests for more money and better staff.

Patients were poorly clothed. They often had no bed linen or medical supplies. The food was bad. The buildings were rotting. The crowding was terrible. Preston encouraged *The Sun* to write about the institutions and promised his cooperation.

The Sun chose a former war correspondent named Howard M. Norton to do the articles. Norton was 38. He had already won a Pulitzer and would someday become Foreign Editor of the paper.

Working with Norton was *The Sun's* chief photographer, Robert F. Kneische, who would describe the assignment as his worst ever.

"I had photographed fire, flood, famine and riot, but never anything as bad as this."

Springfield cooperated completely. Hospital superintendent, Dr. Robert Gardner, and his assistant, Joseph Tomlinson, who people referred to as "Mr. Springfield," welcomed Norton and Kneische, and showed them everything they asked to see and more.

This was opposite the treatment *The Sun* received at Spring Grove, the state's first mental institution, where the aging superintendent did all he could to keep the paper out.

Before publishing the articles, Norton showed them to Dr. Preston. Preston was aghast. He asked *The Sun* not to print them. They printed them anyway. The first appeared on January 1, 1949, only a year and a few months before Helen's arrival. The title was "Maryland's Shame: The Worst Story Ever Told by the Sun-papers."

The articles were brutal. The photographs were viscerally alarming. The public was outraged. The government was forced to react. Soon there were studies and reorganizations and big political battles. And although Springfield did benefit in the end, they felt the Sun had betrayed them by focusing solely and intently on the bad and completely overlooking the good.

About three years later, a man named William Trombley would write a detailed analysis of these articles for *The Sun*.

Trombley quotes one woman as saying, "We had tried for so long to build public confidence in the hospital, to make the public realize that mental hospitals were not horrible. Then Norton destroyed in one day what we had built up over a period of years."

One of the doctors told Trombley, "We poured out information to Norton. We had nothing to hide. We felt we had done our best and that the state hadn't done its share."

In March of 1949, forced into action by the public outcry, the state issued a *Report by the Joint Senate and House Committee to Study the State Mental Hospitals.*

About Spring Grove, they wrote, "The interiors of the institutional buildings are in large part forbidding, unattractive, unsafe, dirty and odorous. In certain buildings the stench was so great as to make several members of the Legislative Committee actually nauseated...

"In some wards there is not sufficient room for anyone to walk between beds, and patients must crawl over the ends in order to get in or out of bed. The so-called 'day rooms' are in fact mere corrals where patients are herded during the daylight hours and are dark, unattractive, uninviting and generally odorous...

"In the disturbed wards...the smell from crowded human bodies was everywhere, and the nauseating stench of urine and fecal matter permeated all the disturbed wards...

"In the old buildings the floors have become so soaked with matter that it would be impossible to remove the odor without removing the entire floors and gutting the buildings."

On the contrary, although they found Springfield overcrowded and understaffed, they wrote, "All buildings and equipment were found to be in exceptionally clean condition. Odors were almost non-existent, except for very slight ones in the disturbed men's day room," and that the employees were "doing a good job...There seemed to be a general feeling of cooperation among the employees, resulting in good morale, and a respect and praise for the administration."

The end result was that despite the tremendous sense of betrayal the articles caused at Springfield, Norton's writing forced the state to react, and eventually money flowed in. But even as they built new buildings and painted old ones and put curtains on windows and replaced old wooden floors with more modern flooring that would mop clean and repel odor, patients continued to pour in.

A Springfield psychiatrist told William Trombley, "We are still so overcrowded and understaffed here that real treatment is only given to a very few. The only cases we are apt to treat are those that catch our eye because of some especially interesting problem."

Helen Starliper of Clear Spring arrived in 1950 with an especially interesting problem.

THE ḦISTORIES

"At no time did that empty smile fade away from her face."

DR. GERTRUDE SONNENFELDT

August 2, Whitey

Exactly a week after Helen was settled into the Hubner Building, the *Hagerstown Morning Herald* announced that Whitey Starliper was running for sheriff.

"A native of the county and lifelong resident of Clear Spring, Whitey has served a number of years as a county constable and thus is familiar with the duties of a law enforcement officer. Married and the father of a large family, he has long been employed as a meat cutter and is presently manager of the meat department of the Self-Service Market at Smithsburg."

As part of the process of bringing a new patient into the system, the hospital took what they referred to as a history, which involved a very detailed discussion with a family member. This was usually done by a social worker and sometimes also a doctor. In Helen's case they did two histories, one with Whitey and one with Lethean.

Some of the questions were of a very specific nature about Helen's life, all the way back to her birth, including questions about breast feeding, menstruation, and sexual development. The hospital must have warned Whitey that they would be asking these questions, because during that week he spoke with Helen's mother.

Annie Small was sickly and over 80 and living with her daughter, Esther. It's not likely Whitey enjoyed speaking with her a week after committing her youngest daughter to a mental institution. But he did, and on August 2, 1950, he met with Beverly Heitmann, the same social worker who had checked Helen in just a couple weeks earlier.

In the history that she wrote afterward, Heitmann described Whitey as a "neatly dressed man of medium build," who "threw his arms and legs about in a nervous gesture" and "discussed his wife's illness with an attitude of detachment, talking strictly regarding factual material and putting in very little feeling. At no time did he indicate that he felt that the illness might have been upsetting to her.

"It was only as he talked of his present difficulties in connection with maintaining a home for the children that he digressed enough to say that he was having a difficult time."

She reported that "the informant spoke of the mother as being very nervous and the entire family is known in the community as being 'queer.' He elaborated on the meaning of 'queerness' by saying that the Shupp family did not associate with other people and seldom even spoke a word to persons who were outside their own family group.

"The informant stated that he first knew the patient when he dated her at the time she was approximately 15 years of age. He did not date her again nor begin to go steady until she was approximately 21 years old.

"Mr. Starliper stated that during their married life they had gotten along quite well. He described his wife as having been babied a great deal by her parents and indicated that she had a very domineering nature and he found it difficult to get along with her unless he gave her her own way. He described her as being meticulous and precise in the care of her house and the children...

"Before the patient became ill, she was described as having been cheerful and pleasant, although somewhat quiet in disposition. She enjoyed the company of others, although she did not enjoy going to movies and parties a great deal.

"For approximately 3 years, Mr. and Mrs. Starliper maintained a home of their own away from either family. Early in 1940 they moved to share a home with Mr. Starliper's mother. Until the patient became ill, each maintained a separate apartment. However, since the patient's illness, Mrs. Starliper, the mother-in-law, has lived with the patient and family and cared for the patient and the children.

"The informant stated that the first change in the patient was noticed in March 1949, approximately one month before the birth of the last child. At that time the patient's walk changed decidedly. He stated that the change in her gait has been constant ever since that time. Mr. Starliper indicated that at times the patient does walk with her normal gait. He felt that the unusual gait is always used whenever she becomes nervous or upset. He illustrated this by pointing out that if you attempted to hand her anything or spoke to her when she was walking about, she would immediately begin using this gait.

"In April 1949, the patient delivered her seventh child...Plans were being made for delivery at the hospital. However, the baby was born approximately one month before it was expected. Mr. Starliper indicated that his wife gave birth to a child following a very short labor...saying that he returned from work late in the evening and found his wife in labor. She had not told her mother-in-law of her condition and he immediately telephoned the doctor and arranged for the person who was to care for his wife to come to the house. Before this person arrived, the child was born. Mrs. Starliper had no complications with the birth and was physically well in about 10 days.

"Approximately one or two months after the baby was born, the changes in speech developed. Mrs. Starliper would attempt to talk and 'yes' or 'no' was just about as much as she could say..."

165

At the end of their conversation, Whitey assured the social worker that when the doctors considered Helen well enough to go home, there would be a home waiting. This was actually an important consideration. It wasn't unusual for a recovered patient to have nowhere to go. As time passed, people were forgotten. They weren't expected to get better and show up years later ready to move right back into life with families that had moved on.

Assuming that Beverly Heitmann accurately described her conversation with Whitey, much of what he said doesn't add up. No one else has ever described Helen as domineering or hard to get along with.

Also interesting is Whitey's description of the Shupps as being "queer" and unsociable and never talking with anyone outside their own family. Hillard Shupp was the goalie on Whitey's soccer team. He was Whitey's friend. He was Helen's friend. He was well-acquainted with both families. Annie's brother Harry Shupp was very close with the family of Helen's brother, Earl.

There was a Shupp at Helen's birthday. There were Shupps at family gatherings and weenie roasts.

Also, it doesn't seem possible that Whitey and Helen lived on their own for three years. The numbers don't work. And when Whitey and Helen moved in with the family in Clear Spring they did not live in a separate apartment. The house was very crowded, and there was no way that Whitey and his family could have had their own space within it. They had one bedroom and that was all.

It's possible that Whitey was misunderstood. It's possible the social worker wrote things down wrong. It's possible that Whitey remembered things wrong. It's also possible that he purposely misled her, because he was embarrassed by his own situation and behavior, or for some other reason. Whatever the case, the history that Beverly Heitmann collected from Whitey seems to be at odds with reality.

August 10, Truth Serum

On August 10, about a week after Whitey's interview, Drs. Taylor and Sonnenfeldt injected 30 cc. of sodium thiopental into one of Helen's blood vessels and conducted what they called a "narcosis interview."

The liquid is mostly known by its brand name, Sodium Pentothal. It's a barbiturate. It's famous from thrillers and detective stories as truth serum.

How it actually works, and how well, is the subject of debate. In Helen's case, it produced results, or at least Dr. Sonnenfeldt felt so.

He reported, "The patient for the most part kept on moving her head from one side to the other and opening her mouth in an infantile orally oriented way as well as displaying the empty smile which we have seen on her in the past. Her answers were prompt and upon encouragement somewhat more articulate.

"The patient was able to convey some bits of information…She comes from a large family, but it seems that she was not a happy member of that family…She got married to Charles when she found herself pregnant by him. She has had seven children…

"She did not want so many children and as far as she is able to put emphasis on her statements said that the last child was not planned and that she does not want any more children. She's not interested in sexual relations, does not want any.

"It appeared that there was some ambivalence in her feelings to her husband. She may have tried to intimate that her husband drinks and sees to it that he has a good time where she had to stay home and look after the children. At no time did that empty smile fade away from her face."

It's very unlikely the hospital knew that Helen was pregnant when she married Whitey. Somehow, she got that across. And everything else she told them was also true. Since they didn't know any of this beforehand, it's unlikely they somehow manipulated her, even unintentionally, to tell them what they wanted or expected to hear. And they don't seem to be interpreting things to further any existing theories they might have had going in.

For instance, when referring to the possibility that Whitey drank and that Helen didn't like it, they wrote, "She may have tried to intimate that her husband drinks and sees to it that he has a good time where she had to stay home and look after the children."

It's hard to say how she could intimate something that complex. They didn't report that Helen said it outright. They left open the possibility that they may have misunderstood. But Dr. Sonnenfeldt also wrote: "…as far as she is able to put emphasis on her statements…"

It sounds as if she was able to speak a bit. How else could she make a statement? How else could she get all these ideas across, while smiling and swinging her head from side to side? And if she could answer these questions, and promptly, if she could make clear that the last baby was unplanned, that she didn't want any more, that Whitey drank, and she had seven children, what does that say about the state of her mind?

How had this drug enabled her to tell complicated and true things to these doctors, when off the drug, she couldn't even talk? Whatever happened and however it worked, it's clear that when Helen arrived at Springfield, she had not completely lost touch with the basic facts of her life and past.

August 13, Lethean

Shortly after Helen's narcosis interview, Lethean met with Dr. Sonnenfeldt. Typically, the doctors didn't leave the hospital grounds to record patient histories, so most likely someone brought her back to Springfield.

Afterwards Dr. Sonnenfeldt wrote, "The patient has been living with her mother-in-law ever since the third child was born…She said that the patient has been neat and clean at all times, but has been a poor cook, and since they're sharing the kitchen anyway, the mother is taking over the cooking, but she never had to assist Helen in keeping the children spotless and the house clean.

"The informant feels that the patient and her husband get along all right. Her son does drink beer and only rarely to excess, and the informant does not feel that the husband's habits have interfered with the patient's happiness. She thinks that they do get along all right and she did not feel that the experience of so many pregnancies in succession has been upsetting to Helen. She, herself, has criticized her son for being responsible for all of these children but he has laughed it off.

"She considers her son a steady and good worker. He has rarely been out of work. At the time when this couple had only two children, they wanted to go into the restaurant business and open up a small place in Clear Spring. Actually, they did not have the money and had to borrow it, but neither one of them were on their toes. They never knew how to plan their expenses and they liked good food and spent a lot on it. Both of them never got up early and it only took a year until they had to give up the business. It was at this time that they moved in with the informant and her husband, who was at that time still alive. The patient's husband never paid his father back what he had given him when he opened up the restaurant.

"The informant had always found her daughter-in-law a lovable person and did not find fault with her. She says she never was an outgoing person, never did much entertaining and had little initiative. She was an indulgent mother.

"The family noted a change in the patient's behavior about three months before the last baby was born. She would stay in bed longer, would be quieter and showed less and less interest in her domestic affairs. The family physician had planned a hospital delivery for her and wanted to sterilize her, but in retrospect the informant feels that the patient did not like the idea of going to a hospital or even was scared. She recalls now that on the evening before the delivery took place, she sent the oldest child to the drugstore for some sanitary napkins and she opened the box and put it aside, and it was the following night the baby girl was born.

"The patient shares a bed with her husband and early in the morning the husband awakened feeling that his wife's knees were shaking."

Lethean says that Helen might have been afraid to go to the hospital. Did Helen somehow know the baby was coming early? Is that why she sent Sonny to the store? Was she planning to deliver the baby alone, without letting anyone know until it was over, so that she wouldn't have to go to the hospital?

Even in Whitey's telling, Helen went into labor without letting anyone else in the house know, including Lethean, who had actually attended many births over the years.

Obviously, she was able to think clearly enough and speak clearly enough to tell Sonny what she wanted from the store and how to get it. And if she could think that clearly, it seems likely she could think clearly enough to know that what she was planning to do, without any assistance, would be awfully hard. She was able to plot. She was able to plan. But was it rational planning?

"OME"

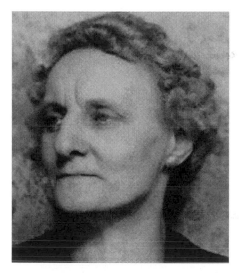

Helen's sister, Nan Seale, was in her early
sixties during Helen's confinement.

The patient sits alone with a vacant but pleasant smile.
One is reminded of a very young child when watching
her walk. Very rarely, she walks quite normally.

DR. BUTTERWORTH, OCTOBER 18, 1950

In August of 1950, the hospital sent Whitey the following form.

I give the Springfield State Hospital permission to use Electro-shock Treatment in the case of Helen Elizabeth Starliper for therapeutic purposes. I give the permission knowing that there are certain dangers in its administration.

That's all. Whitey signed. At the bottom he scrawled, "I cannot pay for these treatments. If at any time I can spare part of it, I will do so."

It was a standard form. It did not mention cost. Electroshock therapy was common and had been practiced in the institution since 1941, but Helen was an unlikely candidate. They knew they wouldn't correct her illness by jolting her brain.

A Dr. Knowles examined her eyes on Friday, August 26. He reported early optic atrophy of a type "often seen in multiple scleroses."

Sometime that same day, Annie Shupp Small passed away at Esther's house. She was 82. In nine years, Helen's nephew, father, brother-in-law, brother, and mother had died. She could not attend the funeral, and it's likely no one ever told her that her mother was dead.

Whitey didn't seem terribly concerned about Helen, and Lethean had no easy way to get in touch, without someone taking her on the long ride out to the hospital. One day she wrote a letter.

Will you please drop me a line & tell me how Helen Starliper is & if you give her the shock treatments and were they any benefit to her? Enclosed find a stamped self-addressed envelope for a reply.

Whitey didn't write any letters with self-addressed stamped envelopes, or without, but he did run for sheriff in the Republican primary. When the votes came in on September 20, he had 531. There were three other candidates. Their totals were 2,274, 1,717, and 1,337. Out of 5,869 votes, Whitey got less than 10 percent.

172

He would never be sheriff, but that October he was elected president of the Washington County Soccer League for the 1950-1951 season. He told the papers he expected it to be a good one.

Also, that October, almost three months after Helen's arrival, Dr. Butterworth presented her case to the hospital's medical and psychiatric staff during their regular staff conference. There were about 15 doctors present, including doctors Salomon and Sonnenfeldt. Dr. Ruth Beyer summarized their conclusion.

"Psychosis associated with organic changes of the central nervous system, multiple sclerosis."

Psychosis is not a disease. It's a condition characterized by a loss of contact with reality. By organic changes, they meant that something physical was causing Helen's symptoms and that this physical thing was affecting Helen's central nervous system. In other words, the disease was slowly severing Helen's connection to the world. They just didn't know precisely how.

During the days of the "Maryland's Shame" articles, one of the doctors said that few patients got individual psychological treatment, unless they presented a case that captured the interest of one of the doctors. Helen captured the interest of a doctor named Parnell.

In February of 1951, after Helen had been in the Hubner Building nearly six months, Dr. Parnell wrote, "She's a woman who has a disease of the brain and is only dying and the best one can do is not make things any harder for her."

He explained that the "psychiatric administration has consisted essentially in trying to make her as comfortable as possible," mixed with a bit of physical therapy. Dr. Parnell encouraged her to walk. He encouraged her to swing her legs out. He did not expect her to improve. But they would do their best to keep her comfortable and moving.

Helen spent most of her time with her legs crossed, her hair mussed, her mouth partly open, sitting in a chair by the automatic water cooler in her room. That also happened to be the chair closest to the bathroom.

Dr. Parnell wrote, "She has partial control of her bladder and bowel excretory functions and usually attempts to walk to the bathroom…Because of her difficulty with ambulation she rarely gets beyond the door of the bathroom unassisted."

The doctor tried speaking with her, but never made any progress. He didn't blame her mind. He blamed "the difficulty she has in the mechanics of verbalization."

He wrote, "She feeds herself with spoon and fork. Sleeping pattern is that she is usually the first patient put to bed by the ward attendant. She tries to cooperate with dressing, but her jerky semi-stiff motor disabilities interfere with the changing of clothes; so far chemical sedations have not been required. She sleeps quietly through the night from 9 PM to 6 AM. On October 25, 1950 she slipped and fell to the floor without doing any bodily damage. In the early part of November 1950, she had tonsillitis and cervical lymph nodes enlarged. This responded fairly well to antibiotics and chemotherapy.

"For the past three or four months she has been living in the medical admission ward with no remarkable changes in herself having been noted. Visitors are rare, coming about once a month for the past three months; a sister and a Mr. Stevens visited on November 19, 1950, and a male cousin visited on December 24, 1950.

"Attitudes expressed by the visitors have been that it was 'terrible that this had to happen to Helen, but there is nothing that anybody, including the doctors, can do about it; and that it is certainly terrible that she is married to a man like Charles Starliper, who is not even interested in visiting her and was a big factor in her present illness.'"

During one of Nan's visits, Helen repeated one word.

"Ome."

She wanted to go home. But Nan couldn't take her home.

Three days after Nan's visit that November, 61 days after Lethean sent her letter with a self-addressed envelope, she received a reply from hospital superintendent Robert Gardner. His office was only a short walk from Helen's ward. Maybe he checked in on her. He was a kind man, who served as superintendent from 1949 to 1961, but the letter offered little in the way of insight or hope and should have at least told Lethean why they had not used shock treatment.

There has been very little change in Helen Starliper. She has not been given any shock treatments. You may visit her on any Sunday or Wednesday afternoon from 2 to 4.

Then came Christmas. Most likely the male cousin who visited on Christmas Eve was Hillard Shupp. Four years earlier in 1946, while stationed with the army of occupation in Japan, Hillard had sent home a letter that appeared in the April 3rd issue of the *Hagerstown Morning Herald*.

By the time Hillard got there, the Japanese had paid terribly for their surprise attack. Millions of their soldiers and sailors and fliers were dead. In a raid on Tokyo in 1945, the allies dropped thousands of incendiary bombs and created a raging fire that incinerated 16,000 square miles and as many as 130,000 Japanese civilians.

Soon after that we hit Hiroshima and then Nagasaki. The two atomic bombs killed 110,000 instantly, and another 75,000 slowly over the weeks to come from burns and the terrible effects of radiation.

One day Hillard visited the ruins of Hiroshima, and then he sent his letter.

"Just how many people perished in that city and just what it actually did to human bodies, I guess no one really knows, because it left no evidence. The outlying districts of the town don't seem to be too badly damaged, but it will be years and years before it will be a city again...if the world knows what's good, science had better stop playing with that invention. Bury it, right away...but now that we have it, it should be instrumental in keeping world peace, or at least we all hope so."

Now Hillard was at Springfield on Christmas Eve. They rolled his cousin out in a chair. He had known her since she was a little girl. Maybe he tried to hold a conversation. Maybe he crouched and looked into her eyes and said, "Helen, it's me, Hillard." And maybe she smiled.

They took her away. Hillard had seen the ruins of Hiroshima. And now his cousin. He drove back to Clear Spring. And then it was Christmas.

The sounds of laughing and singing drifted through hallways and filled the rooms all over Springfield. There was Christmas music and cookies and caroling. The wards were decorated. Helen sat by the water cooler near the bathroom. Maybe Santa peeked in. Maybe Helen smiled bigger than usual.

She had never been away from her children on Christmas before. No one came to see her.

Winter went by and then spring. By the end of Helen's first year in the Hubner Building, she could no longer walk or talk or get herself to the bathroom. Day to day she seemed the same, but as one doctor put it, "progressive deterioration is continuing." He also wrote that Helen seemed to be "quite happy and always smiles when spoken to."

At one point her jaw swelled up. They tried penicillin. They pulled several teeth. Finally, they incised the jaw and "large amounts of yellowish blood-stained pus drained out."

Whitey didn't know any of this. Whitey was a member of the GOP picnic committee. He helped put together a Republican picnic on September 21 at Coffman's clubhouse at Conococheague.

He was still president of the Washington County Soccer League and made the paper in September for his efforts to keep the league viable. There were eight teams, and he hoped to add more.

The paper wrote, "Starliper expressed confidence in the continued operation of the league, pointing out that all indications point to a successful season."

CUSTODIAL CARE

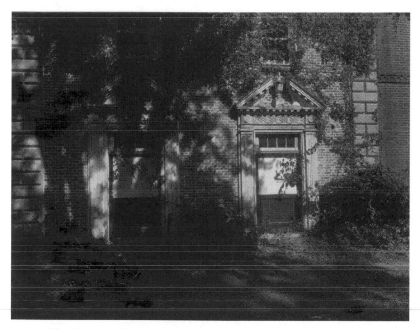

The doors to Cottage 5, September 2020. *Photo by Jack White.*

Will you please tell me just how she is?

MRS. LETHEAN STARLIPER

December 1951

In late December of 1951, Whitey received a letter from the hospital notifying him that Helen had been transferred out of Hubner. From now on, visitors would find her in the Epileptic Colony.

The letter came from Dr. Gardner and concluded, "I wish to ensure you that this transfer has nothing whatsoever to do with the patient's condition or outlook for recovery, as the patients are paroled from the groups on the same basis as from the Hubner Building."

By "paroled" he meant given more freedom and possibly released from the institution. The doctor was saying that Helen was just as likely to be released from the wards in the Hubner Building as from any other, including the building where they were sending her now.

And that was true, in a sense. The transfer had nothing to do with her outlook for recovery, but that's because they had known for quite some time that Helen's outlook for recovery was that she would not.

A Dr. Henry Mead, who the nurses referred to as "Speedy Meady," wrote that "she is younger than those who are usually transferred to Cottage 5, but she is about as helpless as they are. She is transferred for custodial care to the colony."

By custodial care he meant there would be no therapy. They would not try to cure her. They would feed her and dress her and keep her alive and clean until that wasn't necessary.

Dr. Morrell N. Mastin ran the colony. A native of Pennsylvania, Dr. Mastin was about 68 years old. On November 19, he wrote, "This patient was received as a transfer from the Hubner and has been placed on Cottage V where she appears, at this brief visit to be making a fairly good adjustment. The patient will be observed, and if possible, will be placed on a better ward in the near future."

Helen must not have been completely bedridden, because during the early morning hours of New Year's Eve in 1951, while doing her morning rounds, a nurse found Helen leaning over in a chair with her left shoulder pressed against a hot radiator. She suffered first degree burns.

Lethean hadn't heard anything from the hospital, except for Dr. Gardner's brief letter. She couldn't drive. She had no car. Still, she managed to make it to Springfield one more time.

After the visit, she wrote a letter to Dr. Mastin. There's no date on the letter. There's also no "Dear Dr." There's just this.

Dr. Mastin,

I am Helen Starliper's mother-in-law. I was down to see her two weeks ago and I tried to see you at three different times that afternoon but could not find you. What do you think of her condition? I am enclosing a self-addressed envelope. Will you please tell me just how she is?

If Dr. Mastin ever answered, his response didn't make it into the medical records.

THE LAST PICTURE

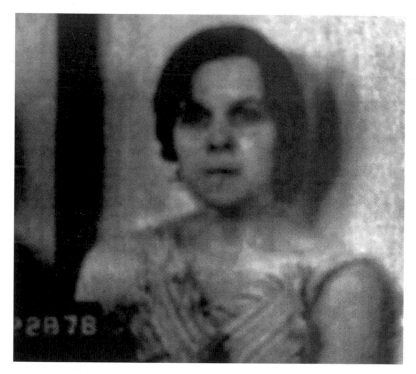

Patient Number 22878

In early December, Helen fell out of bed and cut herself above the left eyebrow. That Christmas was her second away from home. The day after Christmas, one of the nurses noticed a large bruise on Helen's leg. It was a burst vein and not serious. The nurse wrote it down. And then it was 1952.

The war in Korea dragged on. There was a polio epidemic, and medical science was fairly helpless. Over 57,000 were affected with the virus. Over 3,000 died. Many more were paralyzed. Hospitals set up special rooms with iron lung machines and put children inside with just their heads sticking out. The virus paralyzed the muscles in their chests. The machines did the work that their bodies could no longer manage.

Singing in the Rain was a big hit at the movies. Mr. Potato Head made his debut, and the United States exploded its first hydrogen bomb. It was a thousand times more powerful than the ones dropped on Japan.

Apparently, nothing much happened with Helen. There are almost no records for the year. Back in Clear Spring, Sid and Bob worked at the Cohill Orchard every day after school. Whitey drank beer. He played soccer. He cut meat and became friendly with one of the customers who came into the store where he worked. Her name was Gladys.

Hillard Shupp worked for the railroad. That August, someone closed a boxcar door on his hand. The door crushed the hand and cut off Hillard's index finger. Maybe he was still goalie on Whitey's soccer team. Maybe that was the end of his career as a goalie. Maybe he told Whitey about his visit with Helen that Christmas Eve. Maybe he wondered why Whitey never went to see her.

Or maybe no one ever mentioned Helen to Whitey.

Summer passed with windows open and fans blowing. Then came fall and October. The leaves in the courtyard outside her window began to turn, the grass yellowed, and Helen's temperature shot up. Her eyes went glassy. Nurses held her hand and whispered kind words. They dipped sponges in tepid water and bathed her hot skin. They treated the raw patches on her back.

Her fever crossed 105. The nurse reported her smile. And then a bit later, the nurse wrote those mysterious words.

181

"Patient was able to talk."

But that's all she wrote.

"Patient was able to talk."

Maybe it was something as simple as "thank you."

And then it was back to business. Crushed ice, sponge baths, cleaning the bed sores, hitting them with light, taking her pulse, taking her temperature, holding her hand, listening to her hard breaths.

The same nurse who wrote that Helen smiled and was able to talk, also wrote, "In great pain."

On October 6, a different nurse made the following notes.

"No medication given because she could not swallow. Temperature of 105 at 8 a.m. Condition about the same. Breathing fast and heavy."

"10 a.m. coloring improved a little."

"12 p.m. temperature at 103."

"3:55 Deceased—expired at 3:55 p.m. Pronounced dead by Dr. Mastin. Body removed to morgue."

Thelma was 40 when she learned that her aunt and best friend was dead. Genevieve was 37. Shirley was 18 and married and peeling pears at her mother-in-law's house, when Genevieve called and gave her the news. She's still bitter about it.

"My grandmother and my whole family were really upset. They were upset at Whitey. They all blamed him. I remember them saying the doctor said, 'Well, it was having the children all so close together.' And then I'm sure, all the stress on top of it. There was nothing easy. There she was in that house, living with her in-laws all those years. I don't think he ever gave her any money. He never took her anywhere. If she went anywhere, she had to walk.

"Can you imagine her living with seven children that close in age in two rooms, and in there washing. In those days you washed in a wash tub. And she done all her own canning. But she never complained. I don't know how she done it.

"And then the fact that he never went to see her. He never took the children to see her. To keep your children away from their own mother, there's no excuse. What do you think it was like for her that her whole life that she could remember was with her children, and then all of sudden she can't even see you, she can't even say 'hello' to you. That's got to be torture. The family always said your mother died from a broken heart."

In *The Seven Starlipers of Clear Spring*, Sonny wrote, "Most of my brothers and sisters remember little of her. As the oldest, I remember a lot. Mom struggled but could not possibly cope with the unbearable demands and stress of the pace of childbearing, childrearing, and living in the home of her in-laws, where she was not always treated with kindness. Nor could anyone else have coped, as I saw it."

Dr. Mastin wrote the death note.

"The patient just gradually became weaker and showed an elevation in temperature one day and a few days later there was a severe drop."

He listed the official cause of death as "Terminal pneumonia. Psychosis with organic changes of the central nervous system—multiple sclerosis."

The hospital encouraged an autopsy, but Whitey refused.

An obituary reported that "Helen Elizabeth Starliper, wife of Charles Starliper, Clear Spring, died in a Baltimore hospital yesterday afternoon."

They didn't name the hospital.

The hospital took her clothes, whatever those might have been, and left her alone in the morgue in the Hubner basement, her eyes closed, her face covered, lying under a shroud in the dark in a drawer, waiting for someone to take her home.

NOTHING STOPS

Cohill Orchard was just a couple miles south of Clear Spring, a short drive or long walk. Bob and Sid would go there after school and on Saturdays and work for different farmers, baling hay, or whatever else needed doing. They didn't make much, and Sid vaguely remembers his aunt Leila taking their money and stuffing it in peanut butter jars. Each jar had a name on it. Bob, Sid, Betty.

Sid says, "And I remember this one particular day, it was October, and we were sorting apples. I keep questioning myself. How could I be picking up a bushel of apples at nine years old? But it's true. They had a packing shed, and they had a big long conveyer belt, and you would dump apples on the belt, and they would go down the thing and separate. Bob and I were working in the packing house that night. So, we walked home, maybe two miles in the dark."

Aunt Leila was waiting. Leila was the older of Whitey's two sisters and a dominant figure in the family. And now with Helen gone, Leila became Lethean's most important partner in raising Whitey's kids. She was imposing, 31, and not one to mince words.

Sid says, "She was the lady, no doubt about it. She was very direct. If she didn't like you, she'd tell you that. And she was a big influence in raising us kids. She was there all the time. She wasn't a controlling person, but she made sure you got your homework done and ate your meals, and after eating, you did the dishes and did things around the house."

In 1942, she married Homer Vance. At first, they lived with the rest of the family crammed in there with Helen, Whitey, Buck, Sam,

Lethean, and all the kids. Eventually, they moved two doors down and rented a couple of rooms in a nice old house from an older lady who lived by herself. But Leila and Homer were always at dinner, and Leila was a constant presence in the family.

Sid says, "Uncle Homer and Aunt Leila were very good to us. They took us on a vacation to Niagara Falls, which was a big deal for us children. And at some point, Uncle Homer got us a TV and put it in the parlor."

But on this night, when Sid got home dirty and tired from a long day of work and school, Leila was waiting.

"I don't know how, but Bob went to one room, and Aunt Leila took me by the arm and led me to the parlor. She set me down on the sofa, and then she said, 'Sidney, I want to tell you what happened. Your mother's dead.'"

Betty has the printed program from the funeral. It lists all the pall bearers. Jess Hull was one. It was Jess who married Helen Seibert. It was Jess who rented them the building where Helen and Whitey started their restaurant. For years to come, Jess Hull would give Helen's boys their haircuts. Now he helped carry their mother's casket to the grave.

The funeral took place on a Wednesday afternoon at the Rowland Funeral Home in Clear Spring, with school in session right next door. Over 170 people signed the guest book. There were Hulls and Sterlings, Shupps, Starlipers, Sparrows and Smalls, Shirks, Shanks, Shenebecks, Ankeneys, Yeakels, Cloppers, Trumpowers, Robinsons, Kings, Hensons, Brewers.

Sid can't remember any of it. He wonders if he was tall enough to see into the casket. He wonders if he saw his mother dead. He wonders if he saw her face one last time. He doesn't understand why during all that time his mother was gone, no one spoke about her, no one took him to see her.

And then Leila told him she was dead, and he would have to dress up and mourn and watch them lower her into the ground. And she was already a stranger to him.

After the funeral they went home. It was a short walk. Life went on. No one talked about Helen. Whitey went back to doing what he had always done.

"I don't remember seeing much of Daddy," Sid says. "I remember seeing him on the weekends, dressing up and going to the soccer games. He was at the house, but he went to the tavern most nights, and I guess he would come home after we went to bed.

"The sad part is, Mom's dying didn't seem to have any impact on us. Nothing stopped. And I feel terrible about that. I just wish I would have known her better."

Eleven months after the funeral, on September 4, 1953, Whitey married Gladys Feigley and moved to Hagerstown.

LETHIE

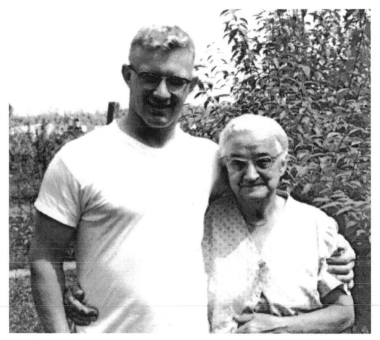

Sonny and Lethean Starliper.

*If God gives any of the human race such a thing as a saint,
He gave us one of his very best.*

SONNY STARLIPER, DECEMBER 2017

187

Helen wasn't coming home. Lethean would raise her kids. She had already raised six of her own. She didn't have any money. It had been several years since her cancer and the colostomy. She had already lived longer than expected, and now she would have to live long enough to get these kids through high school. That would be 15 more years. She set out to do it.

Instead of Sam, Lethie slept with Patsy now. Beverly and Betty slept in a double bed beside them. Nothing much had changed in the house since Helen left. There was still one bathroom upstairs with a sink, a tub, and a toilet. And still no shower.

There was flowery paper on the walls and a collection of not very good furniture. There was a phone and radio and parlor to the right when you came through the front door and a living room to the left, where Lethean liked to sit in a rocking chair. There was the kitchen with a big long table on a floor that wasn't quite level. Leila's husband Homer always sat on the downhill side, and someone was always spilling something. It would roll down toward Homer and he would tilt up the table, and it would roll back the other way.

Behind the kitchen was the room they called the "pack room," filled with all kinds of stuff. There was a cellar with a dirt floor where they stored food for winter.

Sonny Starliper put together a small book about Lethean. Inside he wrote, "No one who did not live there through the years could begin to appreciate the desperate hardship, pain, and poverty that was Grandma's lot in life that she endured for almost 20 years...

"Grandma never had a vacation and never had a day off unless she was too sick to get out of bed. She probably never knew what it was to go out to dinner. She cooked three meals every day, even if all she had to prepare was gravy bread. She and Aunt Leila washed clothes in a wringer washer and hung clothes on the line, even in freezing weather. Grandma was up essentially at dawn, and in winter, came downstairs to a freezing house and made fires in her wood stove and the coal stove in the front room."

But Lethean had her fun. She was a positive person, who made the best of things. In that little book there are pictures of her with a big smile.

She loved playing cards. Sid says, "She would have her very good friends Herbie Sparrow and his wife come, and they would play a game called 'setback.' And I remember that just like yesterday."

Herbie always brought a box of cornflakes. He and his wife slept over and the cornflakes were breakfast.

Lethean had a good support system. There were her daughters. There were Rose and Annie, two sisters about her age, with no husbands or children, who lived right next door.

They enjoyed the little kids. They would all sit out front together in the hot summer nights.

Sid says, "On Saturday night in Clear Spring, people would get their weekly bath. Then they would sit on their front porch or their neighbor's front porch and entertain each other. They cared about one another. There wasn't much money, but there was a lot of love and support and kindness and pleasant times outside during the nice weather."

SISTERS AND BROTHERS

It was quite a collection of characters. Lethean's daughters were sober, hardworking, smart, and responsible. Neither drank. Nellie was the youngest. She was the valedictorian of her high school class in 1945.

At graduation, she gave a speech called "Youth's Part in a Post-War World," and according to the newspaper, all the other kids referred to her as "the heavyweight who was always on top."

After she married Robert Kerfoot in 1947, she moved to Hagerstown and worked at the railroad. She visited Clear Spring often and helped with the kids. Sometimes on Sundays the family ate fried chicken, and Nellie ate with them. Nellie always ate the neck.

Sid says, "At the time I didn't think too much about it. I just figured it was tasty meat. Of course, years later I figured out that she didn't like the chicken neck, she was just making sure everybody else had enough to eat."

Sid's sister Beverly has a strong memory from that time of her Aunt Nellie in a foldup bed in their pack room "crying and crying and crying." Sid believes it was the day they took Helen away.

When she got married, Leila had already been married five years. She worked at a publishing company in Hagerstown. Homer worked at Fairchild.

The brothers were nothing like the sisters. Buck was oldest. He lived his whole life in that house, except during the war. He went into the Army on March 2, 1942, and somehow ended up at what Sid's brother Sonny calls "the meatgrinder of Guadalcanal."

Outside the Army, Buck never held a job, except maybe cutting a neighbor's lawn. He never really made any money. He never owned a car.

When he could scrounge up a few cents, he invariably spent it on something called RWL. Sid's youngest brother Dave says it stands for "run, walk, and lay down."

Sid says, "Whenever he could get 48 cents, he'd go down to the liquor store and get RWL."

Dave says, "He would drink his wine and pass out and leave the empty bottles around. We'd find those empty bottles and we'd fill them with water, and if we could find enough bottles, there was just a little bit of that wine left, and we'd take those and pour them into that water to color it, and he'd come to, and we'd sell it to him for 48 cents. As soon as he'd take a drink he knew right away, and he'd let out a curse.'"

There was constant traffic through the house. At least once a week, Beverly and Betty put down newspaper to keep the floors clean. Buck would tromp right over the papers. The sisters would complain, and Lethean would say, "What am I supposed to do, take him out and shoot him?"

Buck took care of the big garden out back. Potatoes, green beans, sweet corn, tomatoes, onions, squash, lima beans, lettuce, cabbage. There were big grape trees out there, and he took care of them, too. Every November he rounded up a team of friends and butchered two or three pigs in the washhouse out back near the barn.

"Buck was the head butcher," Sid says. "And he would have his buddies help. He would start getting everything ready the day before. There were two large kettles they used for heating the water to boil over the fire. It was still dark in the morning when they started, and they worked all day long. It was a big event for our grandmother, because she depended on all that meat to feed her two families. Nothing went to waste.

"Late in the summer, Grandma and Buck would start canning the vegetables and the fruit. It would take weeks."

Next in line was Whitey. After Whitey came Mason, or "Mace," as they called him. He was the first to go into the Army. He joined in 1940 and spent most of his enlistment with the medical corps at Fort Meade.

After the war Mace might have lived at home a short while, but not long. In fact, no one knows exactly where he lived. They do know where he spent most of his time. That would be the racetrack.

Once, when Sonny asked Mace what he did for a living, Mace answered, "I'm a gambler."

When Dave asked him if he ever worked, Mace said, "I tried it once, but I didn't like it."

Every so often he would show up at the house. Dave says his uncle "would come home either totally broke or with a wad of money that wouldn't even fit in his pants pocket.'"

Mace got married once. Then divorced. Then got married again to the same woman. And then divorced.

Dave says, "He might come and spend three or four days at the house, and then he'd be gone. There were some well-known gamblers around Hagerstown, and he was always mixed in with that group. Everybody just knew that Mace was a gambler and didn't do anything else.

"He was always dressed up. He always wore a white shirt. He would take off his shoes and say how expensive they were. He'd say the leather was so soft you could roll these shoes in a circle."

The youngest of the brothers was Henry, who they called "Tater," as in tater tots. Or perhaps "Tator," for reasons no one knows. He went into the Army Air Corps in December of 1942. Since Mace was in the Medical Corps at Fort Meade, where new soldiers were processed into service, there was a brief time when Henry and Mason were at the same place together.

Apparently, Tater was reluctant to go off and fight for freedom, or even leave the country for the cause. He convinced Mace to help him out with that. They put their heads together and came up with a plan. No one remembers the exact mechanics of the plan, but they do remember that it involved a fake appendectomy, which didn't work out so well.

Tater's hair fell out, and the Army shipped him to India, where he did something with trucks.

He was always looking for ways to make money. At one point, he went into the walnut log business.

"He would go to your back yard," Sid says, "And if he saw a walnut tree, he would be at your front door trying to buy it from you. Right off your lawn."

Sid says, "One of his houses was out on the river above the canal, of all places. There's walnut logs up in the area on the river. This one time, right down close to his house, there was this metal bottom boat sunk in the river with just a small amount sticking out. So, he has this idea he's going to get this boat and fix it up. He's going to cut the logs, float them down the river on this boat, and sell them.

"He gets a tow truck, and we take the cable from the truck clear down across the canal and out into the river, and we hook it on this little ring that was on the bow of the boat. Well, the truck started sliding backward, so we chained the truck to a tree.

"So, I'm down there at the river, and they keep wenching and wenching, and sure enough here comes the boat out of the water, and it comes up on the bank. And then the cable breaks, and the boat shoots back into the river like a submarine so deep we couldn't see it anymore."

Tater married Hazel Murray in January of 1950 and somehow made a lot of money buying and selling land around the canal. No one in the family could figure out how he did it, but he did.

He also drank a lot of whiskey.

Sid says, "I remember him turning yellow, and he got this big belly. He was a normal-sized person, and the doctors told him he had cirrhosis of the liver, and if he would quit, maybe he could live a few years. Couldn't do it."

MOVING ON

*So Buck was there and everybody else in the community.
The doors were never locked, never, and everybody was
always coming and going. All the neighbors.
Everybody slept there at one time or another.
It was like the community center.*

SID STARLIPER

*My brothers and sisters and I can never really know
how much she gave us or what our lives would have
become without her. No one who was not there can ever
really appreciate what she did. Probably all of us were
too naïve to be adequately grateful to her then,
but we understand it all now.*

SONNY STARLIPER

Sid was a Boy Scout. He walked to the Clear Spring schools. On
Sundays, he went to St. John's Church just up the block. He sang in
the choir with Bob and his older sisters. They went to church camp
together and Vacation Bible School and belonged to something called
the "Youth Organization of St. John's Reformed Sunday School."

Ethel Widmyer, who once taught at Sunnyside School, played the
organ at church. She was their choir director and Sunday school
teacher.

Sid's best friend was the minister's grandson, Eugene Hoffman,
who lived two doors down. They played together with Eugene's elec-

195

tric trains, but when the boys were 14 or so, probably about 1957, the authorities took Eugene away. Sid's not sure why. He heard something about Eugene hitting his grandmom. He heard something else about Eugene chasing a girl down the alley.

Sid says, "They put him in a home, and I would go visit him. It was an actual home, where a family would take in troubled children."

Church was a welcome refuge from home, where there were too many people and never enough dollars. Sonny wrote, "Grandma made do with shamefully little money and was unconscionably fussed at by daddy when she practically begged for a little money."

"I remember this one day when I was a teenager," Sid says. "And I came home from school for lunch, and Grandma said, 'Sidney, will you go over to the store and get some bread?' And she carried a little hanky in her apron, and she got in the apron and opened the hanky and there wasn't any money.

"It was just heartbreaking. Fortunately Roger Yeakle, who ran the grocery store, sometimes he would let us get a loaf of bread and put it on the bill, and sometimes he would say, 'Sidney, you've got to get your daddy to pay a little on the bill.'"

In the mid-fifties, Thelma and her husband Dick opened a restaurant called the Chatterbox directly across from the Starliper house and ran it for three years. Sid remembers running over there every time he got a dime or a quarter. Betty worked there. Shirley's brother, Harold Talhelm, held his wedding reception there.

Sid remembers making mayonnaise sandwiches with four slices of bread in winter. He remembers swimming in the local ponds and lakes after church in summer. He remembers their neighbors, Mr. Brewer Gsell and his sister, Erma. They had horses named Queen and Strawberry, and Brewer would plow gardens in Clear Spring with a horse pulling the plow.

Sid's earliest clear memory might be of Mr. Gsell and one of his sheep.

"I will never forget the first day I walked by his barn and he was shearing his sheep. I didn't know what he was doing. He had a table with big wide boards, and on the table, he was holding down one of his sheep with one hand and in his other hand, he had a large pair of scissors or shears. I watched him a very long time. It scared me because sometimes he would cut into the skin. I was so sad that it happened, but I guess it was okay. He would put the wool in feed sacks."

Mr. Gsell was a Mennonite and good friends with Helen and her family. He was one of the wealthiest men in town but didn't believe in banks. He kept his money hidden in the walls of his house.

Sid's favorite memory is Christmas Eve. "We all sang on the junior choir and participated in the nativity scene. On Christmas Eve, we would attend the church service. Afterwards, we would gather in the lower part of the church, which was our Sunday School classrooms. It was such a special time, seeing all your teachers, everybody hanging up their choir robes.

"Mrs. Strite's husband would dress up like Santa Claus and even had a beard. Several of the other teachers would help Santa and pass out our boxes of candy and an orange. I wish I could put into words my feelings about what those two presents meant for us. There was around 12 pieces of candy in each box.

"Then we ran home as fast as we could to show our grandmother what the church gave us. Grandma would go to the pack room and dig out the cookies that she had hidden away. It was hard to go to sleep. We couldn't wait until morning.

"Betty was always the first one awake on Christmas morning. It was still dark, and she would wake the rest of us up. We would hurry down to the parlor. It was so much fun opening the presents and being happy for each other."

The rest of the year, they all worked.

Betty, says, "I used to babysit every kid in Clear Spring. I worked at the grocery store. I worked at the restaurant." It was actually Thelma's restaurant.

Sid played baseball. He played basketball. He played soccer. Clear Spring had a great high school soccer team. At one point they went five years without losing.

"I think we lost the 51st game," he says. "It was a sad thing for Clear Spring when that string was broken."

Sid graduated from Clear Spring High in 1961 with about 40 others. Betty lived with Albert on a farm about five miles down Route 40, and Sid moved in with them. It upset Lethean when he moved out, but she didn't tell him, and he didn't find out till later.

Betty worked at the Potomac Dairy in Hagerstown. Albert laid bricks. They also had a small farm and a lot of pigs.

Sid says, "Each day at the dairy, Betty put the old cottage cheese and milk and everything else in the trunk of her car, and she would bring it home, and Albert and I would open all these boxes and jars of spoiled milk and cottage cheese, or whatever it was, and that's how we fed the pigs. And oh my God, the pigs loved it."

The times were fairly peaceful and prosperous. The Korean War had ended eight years earlier with everything back where it started. Gas cost 27 cents. The Yankees won the World Series. They'd won 16 of the last 32, but this year was special. Roger Maris hit 61 home runs and Mickey Mantle hit 54, while they battled it out to break Babe Ruth's record of 60. Helen was 14 when Ruth set his record. She was dead almost 10 years when Maris broke it on the last day of the season in a game the Yankees won 1-0.

Frank Sinatra was 46. Elvis had two number one hits. No one had heard of the Beatles, Bob Dylan, LSD, hippies, Vietnam, or even the Beach Boys.

Chubby Checker and Lawrence Welk also had number one hits. So did Pat Boone, Ricky Nelson, and Roy Orbison. There were classic songs we still hear today. *Will You Still Love Me Tomorrow* by the Shirelles. *Take Good Care of My Baby*, by Bobby Vee. *Hit the Road Jack*, by Ray Charles.

And Dion warned everyone to "keep away from runaround Sue."

John F. Kennedy was President. He was 43 and the first Catholic to hold the office. The Soviets were our mortal communist enemies. They had H-bombs and transcontinental nuclear missiles. Kids practiced air raid drills in school.

Sid got drafted in 1962, the same year Soviet leader Nikita Khrushchev snuck some missiles into Cuba. Kennedy told him to get them out. Khrushchev did eventually, but only after 13 days when it looked like the world might blow up.

The world didn't blow up, and the Army didn't take Sid, something to do with a bone growth on one of his legs.

In 1963, when he was 45, Mace dropped dead in his white shirt and leather shoes at the racetrack in Charles Town, West Virginia. Two years later, Buck did the same thing, without the horses and fancy shoes, in the house on Main Street. He was 52.

By 1965, Lethean was 79. She had outlived her husband, her daughter-in-law, and two sons. She was into her 18th year since the surgery. The cancer came back, and one Tuesday afternoon, seven months after Buck died, Patsy took her to the Washington County Hospital.

Patsy was 16. She was still in high school and had only recently learned to drive. It was September 22. In an elevator heading up, Lethean told Patsy she had done all she could for them. She'd tried her best. Patsy said it was okay. She couldn't have done more. Everything would be fine.

They stepped out of the elevator, and Lethean had a heart attack. She died there in the hospital.

It had been 15 years since she held Helen's hand in the back of a sheriff's car. Dave was three then. He was 18 now and still home.

Sid was seven then. Now he was 22.

The house emptied out. Patsy moved in with Beverly. Dave moved in with Bob. Whitey was in Hagerstown with Gladys.

Tater bought the house with his second wife, and then he died. He was 47, done in by the whiskey.

Between 1963 and 1967, Lethean and three of her sons passed away. Tater's second wife, Rosa, held on to the house until 1992, when she sold it to Paul Bryan for $54,900. And finally, after 80 years, the house on Main Street in Clear Spring passed completely out of Starliper hands.

DAUGHTERS

Soon after Sid moved in with Betty, her husband Albert got him a job at a masonry company. Sid mixed mud and carried bricks and saved money. He bought a nice 1958 Chevy Impala and promptly took it to Hagerstown and a popular place called Richardson's Drive-In. Richardson's opened in 1948 and lasted till 2008, when chain restaurants and the Great Recession finally did it in.

"It was kind of like that movie, *American Graffiti*," Sid says. "You could park outside, and they would take your order and bring the food out to your car. We would take our hotrod cars and ride around showing off. And of course, somebody would show up with a new car and say how fast it was, and we would say, 'Okay, let's go find out how fast it is.'

"We had a place out in the country where we would go drag racing. We had it marked off, and we would race. And of course, everyone was always trying to make their car faster. We would go to real drag races, too. They had a track there in Hagerstown. And going to the drive-in movie was another thing we did. All the boys would gather up in somebody's car."

They all drank beer, except Sid, who was afraid that if he tasted beer, he would become his father. Eventually, he met a smart, pretty girl. He never really had a girlfriend. It might have been nice and should have been possible. He was an athlete and a nice guy, but he was shy. He didn't attend his prom, or anyone's for that matter. Some of the girls actually decided he was a snob, but that wasn't it.

"We didn't have any money. We didn't have any clothes to dress up in. We didn't have a car to take a girl to the prom," he says.

The girl's name was Karen Runion. Sid told me they met at something called a "hop," which, it seems, was a sort of dance event featuring really good rock 'n roll from the days before the Beatles. At least that's how it looks in *American Graffiti*.

Karen had brown hair, like Sid, and came to Hagerstown from Virginia. When I asked her about meeting Sid at the hop, she laughed out loud.

"A hop? That is hilarious. You would never find Sid at a dance. We met at Richardson's Drive-In. I was studying at a school for medical assistants and lived in a dorm in downtown Hagerstown. We girls would pile in my car and go out to Richardson's. Of course, that's where the guys were.

"He actually dated one of my suite mates, and she introduced us. He was friendly and fun and not cocky. We mostly ran around with our friends. He didn't have money to spend on dates, I'm sure, but that didn't even occur to me. Back then you didn't have to go to fancy restaurants or movies. It was a simple life."

Karen grew up in the Shenandoah Valley of Virginia on a farm, west of a place called Timberville, where maybe 1,500 people lived. Her dad ran a hatchery and raised chickens by the thousands.

Sid was 21 and Karen was 19 when they got married. They had a big wedding, over 100 people, at St. Luke's County Line Church in Shenandoah County, Virginia. Karen wore her sister's wedding dress.

Sid's family made the trip from Clear Spring, except Whitey, who was living with Gladys and her kids. Lethean stood in for Sid's parents. The Reverend Huffman came down from Clear Spring and did the honors.

They had a honeymoon in the mountains in a place called Natural Bridge, Virginia. Sid's first daughter was born in 1968. They named her Helen Elizabeth in honor of Sid's mother, but always called her Beth. Holly Sue came along in 1971, the same year Sid was hired as a carpenter by Miller & Smith, Inc., a builder out of McLean, Virginia. Jill Marie came along in 1977.

There was a son, too, in 1975. They named him Sidney Allen. He had a congenital heart defect and died in Sid's arms at Johns Hopkins Hospital, three days after he was born.

They bought their first house in Funkstown, Maryland, the year Beth was born. Sid built their next house in a development called Crest Valley, east of Hagerstown, the year Jill was born. In 1983, he built them another house on eight acres in that same development.

He worked at Miller & Smith for 45 years, starting as a carpenter and finishing as a production manager.

Karen and Sid divorced in 1995. Karen still goes by Starliper. They're still friends. They still do things together with their daughters and all the grandchildren.

Beth's a middle school principal. Holly teaches elementary music. Jill is a client relations specialist at Bank of America. Sid was a good father.

He coached them. He taught them to play sports. He took them camping in a Plymouth Horizon with some sort of Viking Pop Up camper trailing behind. They headed out west every summer for a two-week vacation. Later they bought a small RV.

Holly says, "For growing up most of his life without his mom, and with a dad who was mostly absent, our dad has been an amazing father. He is by far the most generous man I have ever met.

"In middle school I remember helping him get a 1961 Chevy that was in a field in the middle of nowhere. We towed it home and over the next many months, years, I spent time helping him restore it. I was so happy to be helping."

Jill says, "When I think of my dad, I think of a quiet, gentle soul. And a daredevil. He likes to go against the grain. If the speed limit is 50, he will do 100, if fireworks are prohibited, he lights them, if GPS tells him to go right, he goes left, and if it's Halloween he will give out bananas instead of candy.

"The best memories are driving his car, learning to cut the grass, vacations at the beach with our dog Bear. The most touching thing about my dad is how he has always had my back. Even if the decisions I made weren't the best, he always 100 percent supported me no matter what."

Beth says, "We learned so much from his actions. It was never through a lecture. His actions taught us to have compassion and kindness, as we watched all the hitchhikers he stopped for, all those in need of roadside assistance he stopped for, and the genuine respect he showed to all walks of life."

Beth has a particularly fond memory of the dump truck in the driveway one Saturday morning when she and Holly were heading for basketball practice. Instead of going through his typical Saturday morning routine, which involved scrubbing the garage floor, splitting wood, restoring the old Chevy, and assorted other tasks of that nature, Sid was in the driveway shoveling a giant pile of dirt.

There were no car keys. There was no car. There was just this commercial dump truck sitting there blocking the way.

"Dad, we have to get to basketball practice. The Suburban isn't here."

"Take the dump truck," Sid said. "The keys are inside."

"What? Are you serious?"

"You'll be fine."

Sid kept shoveling. Beth got behind the wheel. The shifter was on the floor. She had never driven a dump truck before, or anything resembling one. They made it to practice on time, then hid the truck so the other girls wouldn't see.

"By example, or by force, my father instilled fearlessness in me," Beth says. "And I love him for that, and for so many reasons."

MIKE

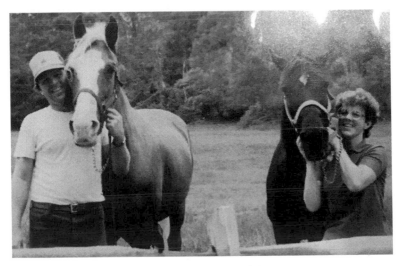

Mike, Charlie, Dee, and Patsy

*During the night I was praying to my mother
to please help me write the book.
About one hour later, Mike came out of nowhere.*

SID STARLIPER, MARCH 2018

*The day of my mother's party, when Mike got up to leave,
I asked him to wait one minute. I handed him the portrait
of Patsy. It was a moment in time that I will never forget.*

SID STARLIPER, AUGUST 2020

The first time I met Mike McKee, he had prostate cancer. He seemed happy and healthy. He didn't say anything about cancer. A few months later, when I met him again, things had changed.

He said, "About a month and a half ago I woke up, and I had a bad stomach pain and a bad pain in my back. I went to the emergency room and I found out I have small intestines cancer." (Mike pronounces it "intesteens.") "And then they done a CAT scan, and I got lung cancer, and two years ago I was diagnosed with prostate cancer.

"They're going to do my lung first. They told me they can take it out. The one I have on my lung is a very aggressive cancer. That's the one they want to get rid of first. The other one, it's not on the inside of my intestines, it's on the outside. It's a very slow growing cancer. That's what my mother has. She's ninety years old."

Mike's mother died early in 2020. Then in late August that year, Sid rode out from Frederick to visit Mike. Mike wasn't home. There was a stranger mowing the lawn. It was one of Mike's friends. Mike was off having chemotherapy, an eight-hour session. There were spots on his liver now and stage 4 cancer.

A couple weeks later, Peachie fell and broke her pelvis. She ended up in the hospital and then a nursing home, too drugged up on painkillers to do more than briefly smile when Sid showed her a proof of the book.

Sid asked if there was any way I could hurry things up. I said I would try.

My first two meetings with Mike were at the Gate House in Sykesville. The last was in the dining room at his house. Mike wore a baseball cap that first time and a pair of straight jeans. He was friendly, and I liked him right away. He knows about horses. He knows about dogs. He once had 27, who he trained to point with their tails in competitions. He built a kennel on his mother's land and kept them there.

He was closing in on 70 when first we met, but seemed younger, and had the most pronounced version of what I've come to recognize as the Clear Spring accent, or Washington County accent, that I've come across. He calls the wash "the warsh." For push he says, "poosh." And of course, there's intesteens.

He has a great way of expressing himself. He once described someone's attitude in the morning (actually it was his wife's) as resembling "a bear with a sore ass." When I met him, he was 12 years on the other side of a hero's slog through hell. And I am not exaggerating.

Mike grew up in Clear Spring, not far up the road from the Starlipers. His grandparents were crop farmers just outside town in a beautiful place called Blair's Valley. He spent his summers with them. He played soccer. He played baseball. He worked on the farm and hung around the old barn behind the Starliper house. In high school and immediately after, he worked at a Sunoco station on evenings and weekends.

The youngest of the Starlipers was a cute little girl named Patsy. Mike never gave her much thought. He was a year ahead of her in school. But then one day when he was a junior, they went on a double date with a guy named Daryl Clopper and a girl who Mike can't remember.

He doesn't remember how he got involved with Patsy, either. She was a cheerleader. He was an athlete. Maybe that was it.

The date went all right. They continued going out on and off, sometimes steadily, but never smoothly.

He says, "I don't know how many times I would take Patsy out back then, and she would get in the car and never say a word to me all evening. And I'd take her home that night and she'd get out and she wouldn't even say 'goodbye.' I called it the 'Starliper pout.'"

Patsy was funny. She was easygoing. She got along with everybody, except Mike. She was also complicated and quirky and powerfully compelled to help other people with their daily needs. Probably to a fault.

And there was something else about her, a secret that Helen passed along. But Mike didn't know anything about that yet. And neither did Patsy.

PATSY

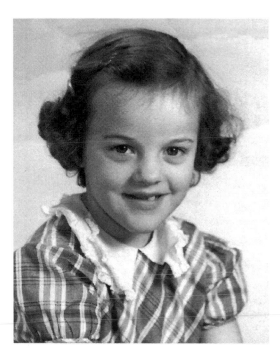

*If she had a problem, Patsy worked her own problem out. She
would never come to me and ask me for help for anything.*

MIKE MCKEE

When Helen died, her youngest daughter was four. Some people
called her Pat. Some called her Patty. Sid calls her Patsy.

In a sense, Patsy never had a mother, but she had her grandmother. She had her Aunts, Leila and Nellie. She had big sisters and brothers and uncles. She grew up surrounded by a family that felt a special sympathy for her. She was the youngest child, the youngest sister, the youngest grandchild. Everyone loved her.

At one point, there was a pigpen out in the barn, and even the pigs loved her. It was her brother Dave's job to slop the hogs, "slop" apparently being a fancy term for feed them. Dave was the youngest of the boys and closest to Patsy in age, with little more than a year and a half between them. Dave would put the dry feed in the trough and mix it up with water.

There was a gate into the pen. Patsy would open the gate and go inside and go from pig to pig scratching their bellies with a corn cob. The pigs liked that quite a bit. And Patsy liked it, too.

Patsy had no memory of Helen. Since no one talked about her, Patsy never talked about her, either, or asked questions.

By the time Sid left home in 1961, the very crowded house had emptied out some. Betty had married Albert. Beverly had married Raymond Stenger, whose father owned Row's Park. All the brothers, except Dave, were gone. Whitey lived in Hagerstown with his new wife and her three kids. Buck was still home and Lethean. The house was less hectic and crowded, and Patsy helped her grandmother take care of it.

Mike says, "Her life was a lot like my life. We worked. We wasn't like city kids. We didn't just come home and didn't have nothing to do. We had chores and work to do. When we was in high school and I was dating her, she'd be ironing and cleaning the kitchen for her grandmother, or always something."

Mike took Patsy to her junior prom, but she went to her senior prom with a boy named Joe Baker. Soon enough, they were back together. But in 1966, right after graduating, Mike got drafted into the Army. He remembers taking a test with his friend Donny at a recruiting place.

"It was multiple choice, and Donny would reach across and color a couple of my boxes in, and I'd reach over and color a couple of his."

Which probably didn't help their scores, but the Army wasn't looking for geniuses, and anyway, Mike switched over to the Air Force. He doesn't remember how, but he was lucky. The Army was most likely a year in Vietnam and a good chance of combat.

The Air Force was four years, and unless you were a pilot of some sort, a much safer job. The Air Force trained Mike as a jet engine mechanic and sent him to an airbase in Dover, Delaware. He came home most weekends, a four-hour drive, to spend time with Patsy.

The US worked out of several airbases in Thailand, and in 1970, they sent Mike to a place called Nakhon Phanom far up in northeast Thailand, right on the border with Laos, a short flight over Laos to North Vietnam, and only 235 miles from Hanoi. He worked mostly on big CH-53 and CH-54 helicopters and stayed until July of 1971.

When Lethean died in 1965, Patsy moved in with Beverly and Raymond on Walnut Point Road about four miles east of Clear Spring. Beverly took over the job of being Patsy's mother, and Raymond bought her a 1957 Chevy.

Sid says, "If you want to know the truth, Patsy was Beverly's kid. Beverly and Raymond took her in and treated her just like they were her parents."

They were strict, too. Years after moving in, when Patsy was in her late twenties, she was still expected home by midnight.

Mike and Patsy continued to date and fight all through his time in Delaware. Before he left for Thailand, he told her to date other guys if she wanted.

If Patsy actually went out with anyone, she didn't tell him, and Mike came through fine. He was 21 when he got home. He proposed, and she accepted. A couple weeks after their engagement, Patsy changed her mind and wouldn't tell him why.

He says, "If she had a problem, Patsy worked her own problem out. She would never come to me and ask me for help for anything.

And it used to make me madder than anything she ever done to me. I could always tell when there was a problem in the family. You could see the look, the Starliper pout. She would never tell me what was going on."

Mike worked at Fairchild at the time, and after breaking up with Patsy, he got into training his 27 bird dogs for competitions. They were English setters and English pointers, and he traveled with them to places like Canada and North Carolina on field trials.

The idea was simple. The dog would spot a target, say a quail or pheasant, and stop and point with its tail. If they broke that vertical point, that was it.

He passed a year and a half without talking to Patsy. He worked. He trained his dogs. He spent time with the horses he kept at his mom's place. He played softball. One day he went into the bathroom of a bar in Clear Spring. By coincidence, the bar was called Helen's, and from the bathroom of Helen's, Mike saw a blue '71 Chevelle go down the alley behind the bar.

Mike was well-acquainted with all Patsy's cars. In 1967, she bought a new dark green Mustang. In '71, she bought the Chevelle he was looking at now.

"And I thought, what in the world would Patsy be going down the alley for? So, the funny thing of it is, she was really doing a lot of work for her church. And that's what she was doing, but she was also checking on me.

"She didn't know I was in the bathroom, but she knew I was at the bar. Anyhow we started crossing each other along our lives, and I just stopped one night, and she pulled up along and asked me how I was getting along, and I said, 'How come you've been following me?' Her eyes got big, and she said, 'What are you talking about?' I started telling her, 'If I go down the street this way, you're going this way. If I cut through the alley, you're over here.' I said, 'I know you've got to be looking.'

"Well, there's another story behind it, too. I really didn't date the girl, but when I went to the bar she was mostly there, and Patsy started playing softball, and this girl played softball. And I think Patsy saw me a couple times with her, and this girl was a little on the wild side, and maybe I'm wrong, but that was always my feeling of why Patsy was watching me. Anyhow, I asked her out."

On their first date nearly two years after Patsy broke their engagement and Mike's heart the first time, they drove to a pretty place called Blair's Valley Lake.

Mike says, "She hurt me so bad that I had no idea of ever asking her to marry me again or anything. But we sat there till five in the morning and talked. I brought up our past history of fighting and laid it on the line. If I come back, there's going to be a guarantee that the family's not going to be part of what I come back to, because that's what the problem was.

"Anyhow, we finally worked things out. I told her I'd like to date and see how things go. I was scared to death to take her home to Beverly that morning."

But he did take her home to Beverly. And they did date. And eventually, sometime around the next Christmas, Mike proposed again.

They were married on September 29, 1979. He was 32. She was 31. They moved into a little property about a mile from Blair's Valley Lake and lived there for the next two and a half years. There were a few rough spots in the beginning, but about six months in, Mike gave her an ultimatum.

"I was working daylight at the time because I was at Fairchild. I would fix supper for her all the time. One evening I fixed fried chicken and everything else. And I had it setting there, and I always figure around five, five-thirty, we'll be eating. Well, eight o'clock she walks in the door. I done cleaned everything up, and I told her flat out right there, that was the last time I'll ever do it. If the family's going to become more important, the way it did here, things are either going to change or I'm going."

Mike didn't elaborate on what was actually happening within the family, and I didn't ask. And after that talk, Mike and Patsy didn't fight much, but there was one more long Starliper pout. A friend told Mike about a horse, and Mike wanted it. For some reason, Mike didn't tell Patsy. He bought a trailer and didn't tell her about that, either. The horse was in Scranton, Pennsylvania, but Mike didn't realize that. He thought he would take a short ride and come back with a nice horse.

Mike says, "Patsy loved animals like you wouldn't believe." So, he hooked up a trailer early one morning and off to Scranton he went to meet the horse.

"He was a great big palomino. He was one of the nicest horses you'd ever want. I wouldn't be afraid to put a six-month old baby up on him. He was really easygoing."

Patsy didn't talk to Mike for two weeks.

Eventually, they moved to a home out in the country closer to Clear Spring. The house needed a lot of work, but it had a barn, and the surroundings were beautiful, with a stream running alongside their yard and Fairview mountain, with its trees heading up into the sky, right there in front of them, nothing between them and it, but a bit of distance. They thought it would be a nice place to keep their horses and raise a family. But it turns out both had medical problems that made a family impossible. At least the type with children.

So, it would be Mike and Patsy and the animals. Patsy made Mike give up the dogs, but there were cats and horses. They named the first horse Charlie. Patsy loved Charlie. They fixed up the house and barn. They bought a Tennessee walker named Dee to keep Charlie company. They boarded two other horses for a friend.

When Charlie had problems with his hooves and could hardly walk, they took him to a place in Leesburg, Virginia, for treatment. The boarding bill alone cost $5,000.

214

"You wouldn't believe how much hoof they cut off," Mike says. "I wanted to have him put down, but Patsy wouldn't let me. She loved that horse with a passion. Probably takes an hour and a half, and every day she went to see that horse, three hours of driving, every day."

Eventually, they moved the horse to an expert in Frederick closer to home. Patsy visited Charlie every day for three months till he finally came home. She would ride him up along the mountains. One day she fell off and hit her head.

Mike says, "They took her to Washington County Hospital, and she had a pretty mild concussion. They kept her overnight, and all the time at the hospital, she kept crying and saying, 'Don't let Mike kill the horse. Don't let Mike kill the horse.' Well, I didn't kill the horse, and I can guarantee you I'd be looking for another home if I did."

Mike liked Fairchild. He started out as a sheet metal mechanic. But soon, the company started laying people off on their way to eventually shutting down. Mike was one of them. And there weren't many other good places in the area to work.

"When I got laid off from there," he says, "I had no choice but to...well I had a choice, but I became a correctional officer."

He despised it, not necessarily the work, but the people he worked for, the bosses above him. It was all bad in one way or another.

"When you work all your life, and then you go as a correctional officer, and you walk out of the jail, you don't see anything that you accomplish. I had a hard time with that."

The prison was called the Maryland Correctional Institute, off Route 70, about 20 miles before Clear Spring, heading up from Frederick, and that's where Mike worked the next 25 years.

Patsy worked at Potomac Edison, where she'd started right out of high school. Originally, she did clerical work in the legal department, but eventually she became a paralegal, working mostly on what they referred to as rate cases.

It was a friendly place where everyone smiled and said "hi" out in the hallways. Even the executives. After she'd been there a few years, Patsy made good friends with another young woman named Jane Fisher.

One day, I called Jane from my father's house in Philadelphia. Jane was in Hagerstown when we talked. She was very fond of Patsy and had to stop now and then to cry. She said Patsy was probably the nicest of all those nice people at Potomac Edison.

"She had a very funny sense of humor. And in legal, Patsy had a very demanding job. There were a lot of deadlines, but I never saw her in a bad mood. She was always smiling, always laughing. And she was always doing something for somebody else.

"'I gotta run here after work. I gotta do this. I gotta do that.' I'm like, 'Holy hell, Pat.' But it was just nothing to her."

Mike says, "Patsy was always getting stuff for Bev, well other people in Clear Spring, too. That was her thing. She was always giving to people. Even my mother. If she stopped and got donuts for herself, she got for Bev, she got for Mom.

"She did that every night. That's the way our marriage was. There was never a set time you sat down to eat. That was Patsy. You just couldn't change her."

"She was always helping somebody," Sid says. "And she was always late. She went to get somebody's prescription. She went to get somebody groceries."

Mike says, "It would be time to go wherever we had to go, and that's when Patsy would decide to wash the car."

In a way, when Mike started at the prison it helped their marriage. Patsy could do all the helping of other people she wanted, and Mike wasn't there to notice. But there was still the problem of the red velvet cakes. Patsy really liked making these cakes.

"She's up at midnight making red velvet cakes when I come home from work," Mike says. "She'd be up till one o'clock, two in the morning. And she was no morning person. In the morning, you didn't say 'hi' to her, you didn't say nothing."

Mike worked at the prison from four to midnight. Patsy worked daylight hours at Potomac Edison, then ran around helping people and making red velvet cakes. They took care of their horses and cats. Eventually, they would meet up at home.

Jane says, "They lived in a very nice house down a country road with a black railing, a beautiful two-story house. You passed the barn. The horses would be out as you'd drive down the lane, and they would come to the fence and look at you, and I would usually wind down my windows and talk to them. Patsy would feed them and get them fresh water. She did a lot of work."

In 1996, Potomac Edison performed what they called a "downsizing," and lots of people lost their jobs. They reorganized, too, and Jane and Patsy ended up in the same department for the first time and became very close.

Jane says, "One of the men gave her the nickname Peppermint Patty. I always knew that Pat was a super-nice person, but after I got to work with her and got to know her, I realized how funny she was and how nice she was. I never heard her talk nasty about anybody. And she just dearly loved Mike. And I know he loved her.

"And she was just always doing stuff for other people. Whenever we had a party for any occasion, we would ask her to make her red velvet cake. It was really delicious.

"And after work, Pat was like, 'Oh I gotta go to Walmart. I gotta stop here. I gotta stop there.' And of course, she had the horses.

"Pat's cubicle was kind of away from anybody else's cubicle and she could play her radio. She would play it low. When the radio stations would begin playing the Christmas songs, she would come over and she would say, 'You have to come listen to this song, I just love this song.'

"It was like a pop rock song, kinda like 'Rockin' Around the Christmas Tree.' Any time it would come on, she would call me, and

217

I would run over to her cubicle. And it was kind of catchy. It was 'All I Want for Christmas Is You.'

"It's not the one sung by Mariah Carey. I liked it so much I had to find out who was singing that, and it was this group I never heard of called Vince Vance and the Valiants. Pat dearly loved it. Every year she would say 'They're playing that song again.'"

Jane and Patsy took a couple trips together for work, and that's when Patsy talked about things she never talked about with Mike, or anyone in her family.

Jane says, "She talked constantly about her family. She loved her brothers and sisters. She told me she always felt cheated that she never had a mom. She was always sad that she never knew her mother. It always seemed so unfair. She talked about her mother a lot."

PATSY THROWS THE BOOK

*Patsy had classes for work, and she had to go into trig and
stuff, and I'll never forget, she was sitting there trying to
figure something out, and then she threw the book. And
that's when I knew something was drastically wrong.*

MIKE MCKEE

After a rough start, it turned into a good marriage. Then, 17 years in,
Patsy found a lump. It was February of 2000 when they did the lumpectomy and removed the cancer from her left breast. They followed
the procedure with seven weeks of radiation. They began the radiation treatments on March 13. In late March, they started her on
Tamoxifen, a relatively new drug approved in 1998 to treat breast
cancer and help prevent its recurrence after surgery.

Everything seemed to go well. It was stage one. There were no
signs of cancer after the treatment. But Patsy couldn't get her energy
back. She was tired all the time. Sometimes at work, she didn't think
she could make it through the day. Thinking it might be the
Tamoxifen, she stopped taking it. But nothing changed. She was still
tired all the time, and they went on thinking it had something to do
with the cancer or the radiation or the drugs.

But there was something else. About a month earlier, probably
sometime in July of 2001, both Betty's husband and Beverly's noticed
something strange about Patsy's walk.

"She was walking up the steps," Mike says, "And instead of lifting her left foot up, she kind of just drug it."

Mike hadn't noticed. Neither had Patsy. Or at least she hadn't mentioned. No one jumped to any conclusions or made any connections with Patsy's mother. Patsy was 49. Helen was 36 and a few months into Patsy's pregnancy when she began dragging her own foot. And Patsy didn't know about that. And neither did Mike or anyone else, except Aunt Leila, who was 80 years old.

That September, Patsy went with Beverly to see Dr. Joseph Cofrancesco, Jr., at Johns Hopkins in Baltimore about her constant fatigue. At first, they talked about sleeping problems. And then Beverly told the doctor about the walking.

Afterward, the doctor wrote, "It seems the patient has been 'walking funny,' per the sister. The patient describes that when she climbs down the stairs, she has to hold on because of the sense of unsteadiness…"

The doctor described her as quiet and cooperative. He mentioned numbness in her feet. He commented on her walk and that "she did have an unusual gait in that she seemed to be somewhat 'slow' in her left leg."

There were other symptoms, but nothing that added to up to something immediately recognizable. He wrote that "diagnosis is illusive" and that "it was truly a pleasure meeting Ms. McKee."

His strategy was to wait, have Patsy undergo an MRI, and then talk again. But the problem wasn't just fatigue or trouble walking or a sense of dizziness.

Jane says, "I remember Patsy started noticing things. New things that she had to learn, all of a sudden became hard for her. The things she already knew, she never forgot, but Debbie Bechtel, she was the secretary, Debbie and I would kind of help Pat with the newer stuff.

"Actually, we were covering for her a little bit. And the bosses knew, and they were like, 'fine, we understand completely.' She was still doing work, but the newer stuff was difficult for her, and that's how she realized something was wrong. She would come over to my cubicle, especially when she would go to the doctors. She was getting worried, because no one could quite figure it out."

Mike says, "Patsy had to have classes for work, and she had to go into trig and stuff, and I'll never forget, she was sitting there one day trying to figure something out, and then she threw the book. And that's when I knew something was really drastically wrong. Not because she threw the book, but because she couldn't get what she was learning."

On September 24, Patsy signed a form granting something called Durable Power of Attorney to Mike and to her youngest brother, Dave. A week later, she went in for her first MRI at Hopkins.

MRI stands for magnetic resonance imaging. It's an amazing invention that came into widespread use during the eighties and revolutionized the way doctors peer inside a patient's body. The process relies on a giant tube with a bed that slides the patient in and out of the tube. The system uses two large magnets, radio waves, and software to work a sort of magic on the cells and derive detailed cross-sectional pictures from inside the body. With an MRI, doctors could analyze Patsy's brain in great detail on a computer screen.

"Me and Sonny and them took her down to Johns Hopkins," Mike says. "They had to anchor Patsy's head in place. She wasn't allowed to move. She laid two hours and 45 minutes with her head clamped in a MRI. Two hours and 45 minutes, and I was right there beside her."

Doctors in Frederick blamed her exhaustion on sleep apnea. They told her she wasn't sleeping. She didn't agree but went through some testing just the same. The test involved sleeping under observation at a study center. She went through it once with no conclusion. They tried again, but this time she called Mike at 3 a.m. and said, "Come down here and get me out."

Her speech kept slowing down. She walked slower. She drove slower. At one point, Mike's mother told him Patsy was driving away from home at 10 or 15 miles an hour on her way to work. He had no idea, and after that, he drove her.

"Her whole body just started to deteriorate," Mike says. "Her mind, her mobility, her arms. But she never complained. That was her makeup. Even when she had the breast cancer. I tried to talk with her about it, but she wouldn't talk about her problems."

Somehow, Sid's brother Sonny knew Dr. Richard Johnson, the director of the department of neurology at Johns Hopkins University in Baltimore and chief neurologist at the Johns Hopkins Hospital. He was one of the top experts in the field in one of the best hospitals in the world. Dr. Johnson knew Charlie well enough to refer to him by his nickname, "Sonny."

The following January, they got in to see Dr. Johnson in his office at Hopkins. Johnson had silver hair. He was world renowned. He had been practicing medicine and scientific research at the highest levels all his life. He was an expert on viral infections of the nervous system, on multiple sclerosis, and neurological disease. He'd worked in places like Iran, Germany, Peru, and Thailand. He won awards. He edited books. He wrote a book. He published hundreds of articles.

They met with him on January 23, 2003. By now, Patsy had undergone two MRIs, two angiograms, which involved sending a tiny camera up through her arteries, and several other tests. Dr. Johnson had all the results, and after their visit, he wrote, "This is a complex case of leukoencephalopathy."

Leukoencephalopathy.

It was a big, long, complicated word, hard to spell and hard to say, until you got the hang of it. No one in Patsy's family had ever heard of it, but soon they could all say it and struggled to understand it.

The word breaks down into three smaller words from Greek: "leuko" meaning white, "encephalo" referring to the brain, and "pathy" meaning disease. Dr. Johnson was talking about a disease of the white matter in Patsy's brain.

Most everyone has heard of gray matter, but the brain contains an equal amount of white matter. Gray matter does the processing. White matter enables the gray matter to send and receive signals. Without healthy white matter, the brain can no longer coordinate all the complex functions that keep the body alive and the brain aware. As the white matter deteriorates, simple tasks become increasingly more difficult, until eventually a woman begins dragging her leg and discovers that walking doesn't come naturally. Walking is complex. And it doesn't matter if your legs and muscles and tendons and all the rest are fine. If something goes wrong in the brain, you still can't walk.

The brain cells carry information to their various destinations across the body on incredibly thin cables called axons. For these signals to travel correctly, a coating of a substance called myelin must insulate the axons. This myelin has a white appearance and acts like the insulating material on wires, sort of like speaker wire. If the myelin deteriorates in some way, signals are disrupted, and the music becomes faint and garbled and eventually stops.

For Patsy, the music was slowly stopping.

At Springfield, they diagnosed Helen with a disease of the central nervous system. The central nervous system includes the brain and the spinal cord. There's also a peripheral nervous system, consisting of all the nerves outside the central nervous system that connect it to the rest of our bodies, to our skin, our limbs, and muscles and organs. Signals between the brain and body travel in both directions up and down the spinal cord.

For the most part, the doctors at Springfield agreed that something was harming Helen's central nervous system. They also mostly agreed that she had multiple sclerosis.

No one knows what causes multiple sclerosis, but they do know that when a person has it, their body's immune system begins attacking the myelin around nerve cells. This leaves scarring in the areas attacked.

Multiple sclerosis is a demyelinating disease. This type of disease attacks the white matter. There is another category of disease called the leukodystrophies. On their website, the National Organization of Rare Diseases (NORD) defines these diseases this way: "Leukodystrophies are a group of rare, progressive, metabolic, genetic diseases that affect the brain, spinal cord and often the peripheral nerves. Each type of leukodystrophy is caused by a specific gene abnormality that leads to abnormal development or destruction of the white matter (myelin sheath) of the brain. The myelin sheath is the protective covering of the nerve and nerves can't function normally without it. Each type of leukodystrophy affects a different part of the myelin sheath, leading to a range of neurological problems."

The visible symptoms of both demyelinating diseases and the various leukodystrophies can be very similar. Based on their observations and understanding, the doctors at Springfield came to a sensible conclusion. But they didn't have MRIs or any other good way to see what was actually happening inside Helen's head. Although the first of the leukodystrophies was discovered early in the 20th century, no one at the hospital ever mentioned leukodystrophy in reference to Helen.

Dr. Johnson wrote, "Her mother died of what was called multiple sclerosis. She became sick at 35 when the patient was a tiny child and died 4 years later in a psychiatric hospital. It was a relatively sudden onset and at about two years after the onset of the disease she was sufficiently deranged mentally that she had to be institutionalized and died two years later. This would be a remarkably fulminant course for multiple sclerosis."

Dr. Johnson was an expert in MS. By "remarkably fulminant" he meant that whatever had hit Helen had struck too suddenly and moved too quickly, going from detection to death in four or five years. He doubted that multiple sclerosis would behave that way.

Compared to the doctors at Springfield, Dr. Johnson had a mountain of information to work with. He had the information about Helen. He had another 55 years of medical knowledge and technical advancement. He had better machines, better tests, better data, more experience with diseases like these, and a detailed knowledge of how they worked, how they differed from one another, and what they could do to a person.

And of course, he could do something the staff at Springfield couldn't dream of doing. He could see three-dimensional images from inside Patsy's brain. But with all those advantages, he was no more capable of curing Patsy than Springfield was of curing her mother.

He gave her various tests. He noted that "at times she looked bewildered" and had to turn to Sonny for help answering questions. He asked her to subtract seven from 100 and keep going to see how far she could get. She couldn't get past 86. He asked her to spell "world" backward. She dropped the "O."

But mostly he said things that only doctors would understand. He spoke of a "rather startling erythema from the mid-calf down." He said that her "feet and the lower parts of her legs are hot and swollen to mid-calf with a heavy edema more notable on the left than the right."

He spoke of "normal optic fundi," and a "mild right facial palsy." He spoke of mild weakness, brisk deep tendon reflexes, and "no obvious sensory abnormality and no cerebral ataxia."

Patsy's white matter was definitely damaged, but the doctor couldn't decide whether she was suffering from a demyelinating disease, such as MS, or maybe another disease called "progressive multifocal leukoencephalopathy (PML)," or some sort of vascular disease. There were other possibilities, too. He ordered tests for HIV I, which would turn out negative, as expected, and for a rare disease known as CADASIL.

They went home. They printed out articles about PML. They learned what they could about CADASIL. They read about leukoencephalopathy. They worried. They waited for calls, for appointments, for test results and answers. They wrote letters and emails. They left messages and waited for responses. There was an awful lot of waiting, terribly worried waiting, and then, finally, the appointments, the disrupted days, the long drives, the sitting in waiting rooms with groups of other anxious people, nervous and frustrated and confused, snacking on bad food, or not eating at all, watching bad TV, and waiting and thinking and pacing, bored and scared and hating it all.

It was hard to get appointments with Dr. Johnson. And when they finally got an appointment, they would always be on time, or early, and then wait forever, or so it seemed, before they finally got in.

At one point, Mike got the doctor on the phone and said Patsy was going downhill. The doctor called Patsy. She told him she was fine. Things hadn't changed that much. The doctor wasn't sure who to believe, but then on May 15, 2002, he got his answer when Patsy shuffled into his office with Sonny and Mike.

He hadn't seen her in four months and knew immediately that she was the one being dishonest, either intentionally or not.

After the visit, he wrote, "It is very clear that she has been becoming worse, that there is a greater evidence of weakness of the left side, particularly in the left hand, that her memory has worsened and she is becoming increasingly impatient, and that she is having more difficulty doing simple tasks around the house even though she has continued to work about 30 hours to over 30 hours a week at her job."

He wrote that Patsy had "remarkably little insight" about her condition and that she "does minimize all findings." He said she had "trouble remembering very simple things from the recent past. She walks with a very hesitant gait, almost shuffling, and takes many steps to turn."

He requested a psychiatric evaluation, and on August 23, 2002, they met with a neuropsychologist named Karen Bolla at Hopkins Bayview Medical Center in Baltimore. By the time they saw Dr. Bolla, Patsy was having a tough time walking. She had trouble controlling her left hand, she was dizzy, constantly fatigued, could hardly sleep, and was easily confused. She put things down and couldn't remember where she put them. She had trouble judging the passing of time.

And like Helen in 1949, she lost interest in the rudimentary requirements of daily life. She didn't cook anymore or clean and really did very little at all except sometimes help harvest the corn on their land.

Eventually, she couldn't dress herself without Mike's help. She couldn't learn the new stuff at work and was even having trouble typing and filing, but yet she managed to keep working 30 hours a week.

After the visit, Dr. Bolla wrote, "Mrs. McKee's a right-handed, Caucasian woman, who was early for her appointment, which she attended with her family. Mrs. McKee was dressed neatly and casually. Her gait was slow, unsteady, and shuffling. Her affect was rather flat, with minimal spontaneous speech noted.

"When answering questions, her speech was fluent and goal directed. However, she sometimes began a response but failed to complete it. Sometimes Mrs. McKee failed to respond until questions had been asked several times. However, once she initiated a verbal response her speech was normal in rate. She often experienced difficulty grasping task concepts as well as remaining on task. Therefore, she required redirection to task on several occasions.

"Mrs. McKee was oriented to person and time. Although she knew the correct city, state, and floor, she reported the hospital's name to be 'eBay medical Center.'

"Mrs. McKee experienced difficulties in the areas of expressive language, learning and memory, organization and planning, attention, executive functions, reaction time, and motor performance with the right-hand."

All told, the results were terrible.

It remained difficult to see Dr. Johnson, but they were finally able to schedule a follow-up. They all headed out to Baltimore one more time. By now they were starved for information and maybe a dash of hope, but the doctor didn't have that much to offer.

Afterward, he wrote, "It is rather extraordinary to me that she is continuing to work, although she has been offered early retirement." And, "She has a progressive downhill disease of several years duration."

Finally, he noted, "I talked with her brother, sister, and her husband today, and I think all agree that the time for a definitive diagnosis and biopsy is upon us. I told her that I had talked with Dr. Rafael Tamargo regarding a biopsy, and that I will go ahead and arrange this. I will be in contact with the family as soon as I have talked with Dr. Tamargo."

There was another layoff at work. This time, anyone over 50 could voluntarily take some sort of retirement package. Jane and Patsy both took it.

THE PURPLE WALL

He told me he never run into a brain that tough.

MIKE MCKEE

Biopsy isn't a word you want to hear. In Patsy's case, it was an especially dire prospect. Her doctors felt they couldn't learn anything more by sliding her into tubes or sending cameras through her veins. If they wanted more information, they'd have to drill through her skull.

The doctor who would do the drilling was Rafael Tamargo. They met him in the morning of September 17, 2002, in his office on the 5th floor of the Hopkins Outpatient Clinic on North Caroline Street in Baltimore. They arrived early, as directed, and brought with them, also as directed, originals of all the X-rays, MRI scans, myelograms, angiograms, and other scans, grams, documents, numbers, forms, IDs, and questionnaires they'd accumulated over the previous months. Duplicates wouldn't do.

Dr. Tamargo had graying hair, a big graying moustache, the slight accent of someone who grew up speaking Spanish, and a friendliness and concern in his eyes that immediately made Mike feel better. His middle name was Jesus, and Mike says Dr. Tamargo was the nicest doctor he had ever met.

Dr. Tamargo was also compassionate and honest. He wanted them to understand that he considered Patsy's prognosis "dismal." He told them any news they got from the biopsy wasn't likely to be good and that there was only a 20 percent chance the biopsy would tell them anything. They would have to weigh that against the ten percent chance something would go wrong, including the possibility that Patsy might not survive.

Patsy was increasingly confused. Her memory was failing, but she knew what was happening. She understood the risks and decided to take them. No one tried to talk her out of it. No one wanted to believe she was doomed. And if the biopsy did kill her, well, not having the biopsy would kill her, too. The biopsy offered faint hope, but faint hope was better than no hope.

Two weeks before the biopsy, Patsy fell while taking a single step up the stairs in her house. When Mike got to her, she couldn't remember what happened. It was the third time she'd passed out.

On October 18, 2002, with Mike behind the wheel, Patsy, Beverly, and Sonny, with his wife, Lois, headed for Baltimore. They were told to be there at 4:30 a.m., and this wasn't one of those occasions when Patsy would decide to wash the car first.

They carried a rough computer-printed drawing of the clinic, a sort of primitive map made of lines and squares and various rectangles that said things like "Oncology," "Maryland Hospital Laundry," "Radiology," "Children's Center." There was a big black arrow pointing to a spot between a couple of the boxes.

It said, "We are here." And someone had printed, "Follow signs to S-7. Osler 7th floor. Same day surgery. Use Halsted elevators to get to 7th floor. Get off elevators and go left. Then look for purple wall."

Osler was circled with a thick black marker. Both Osler and Halsted were important doctors from Hopkins' early past.

At this point, Patsy could still walk, but she shuffled and had to concentrate. They got off the elevator and followed the directions toward the purple wall. They went left at the purple wall and soon found the doctor.

Patsy signed a form that said, "I hereby give my consent and authorize Doctor Rafael Jesus Tamargo and Associates of the Johns

Hopkins Hospital to perform the following operation or other procedure."

There was a line beneath that. Printed above the line were the words, "Right frontal craniotomy for brain biopsy."

The Johns Hopkins' website defines a craniotomy as the "surgical removal of part of the bone from the skull to expose the brain. Specialized tools are used to remove the section of bone called the bone flap. The bone flap is temporarily removed, then replaced after the brain surgery has been done."

So, Patsy signed the form granting Dr. Tamargo the right to temporarily remove a piece of her skull so that he could get at her brain.

She also reviewed a supplemental consent form that listed the risks of the operation. There was a 10 percent chance one of these things, or some combination, would happen.

"Bleeding, infection, pain, re-operation, numbness, weakness, paralysis, mental status changes, dementia, blindness, visual deterioration, double vision, decreased hearing, hearing loss, seizures, stroke, heart attack, blood clots, pulmonary embolism, cerebrospinal fluid leak, coma, vegetative state, death."

She signed that one, too.

The diagnosis was "neurodegenerative disorder of the brain." Their intent was to harvest brain tissue and multiple microbiology specimens.

Mike says that once all the paperwork was finished, "they took her into a prep room where you had to change into a gown and all that stuff, and I went back in there. Then when he took her into the operating room, we went with her so far, but not all the way into the operating room."

Patsy was in the hands of Dr. Tamargo and a team of other highly skilled specialists. They were going to put Patsy's head in a special holder, open her skull, and snip out bits of brain. And Mike, Charlie, Lois, and Beverly were going to wait.

Hours passed.

"We was all scared," Mike says. "I thought something happened or something was wrong. It was only supposed to take so long, and he was only supposed to do the front part of her brain. We all got on the panic side, I guess."

And then Mike heard his name over the speakers.

"It scared me to death."

Dr. Tamargo met him outside the operating room and told him they were having trouble getting all the brain tissue they wanted.

Mike says, "He apologized to me for taking so long. The tissue of Patsy's brain was the toughest he ever encountered. He told me he never run into a brain that tough. He said it was tougher than leather, because that's what the disease does to the brain."

Mike went back to waiting. The doctors got back to work. They followed the damaged tissue from the front of the brain and then toward the back, trying to find the end point. A neurologist named Dr. Carlos Pardo-Villamazar took some brain tissue and microbiology specimens. And finally, at least five hours after they started, they put Patsy's head back together.

Dr. Tamargo recorded the procedure.

"The bone flap was secured with Leibinger plates. The area was thoroughly irrigated...The skin edges were approximated with staples. The patient was reversed and extubated without difficulty and was transferred to the NCCU with her baseline neurological problems."

They put what they'd collected from Patsy's brain in a saline solution and labeled it, "McKee, Patricia—brain tissue."

There were seven fragments of "brain tissue, cerebral matter, and white matter," which they intended to test for mycobacteria, virus, fungi, and any other sort of living things that might have been responsible for tearing up Patsy's brain.

And it all came back negative. No living thing was doing the damage. At the bottom of the form reporting the results, there was a note that said, "There is prominent degeneration of the white matter with gliosis and fragmented axons."

This was important information and more very bad news.

Dr. Tamargo called Patsy at home shortly after she returned from the hospital. He called on one or two other occasions to check on her. Mike liked hearing from him.

A month after the operation, they visited him again. The doctor wrote, "On examination, the wound healed nicely with an excellent cosmetic result. Her neurological condition, however, continues to deteriorate, and now it appears to be affecting the right side.

"I once again had an extended discussion with Ms. McKee and her family concerning the dismal prognosis concerning the situation. Although they do not have a specific follow-up appointment with me and neurosurgery, I asked them to call with any questions or concerns. They have a follow-up with Dr. Richard Johnson."

Shortly afterward, they saw Dr. Johnson for the last time. He still didn't know precisely what was wrong. He described it as "a degenerative process of undefined nature" and noted that she "continues to have a relatively slow progressive downhill course."

He was struck by her "bland smile and affable appearance." He noted that it took her about a dozen steps to get around…"

Aunt Leila was with them. She told the doctor that Patsy looked now exactly like Patsy's mother looked when they took her to Springfield five decades ago.

The doctor wrote, "There was no clear-cut diagnosis made on her mother, but I am certainly suspicious that this is a familial form of a neurodegenerative disease."

Dr. Johnson told Mike that Patsy had less than 18 months to live. There was nothing more he could do.

THE NATURE OF THE BEAST

One day Mike was lying beside Patsy in bed, when she began flailing about. Her mouth filled with foam. Her eyes rolled up in her head. He was terrified. He called 911. It was her first seizure. They gave her medicine for it, and that helped. At one point, they tried another medicine, he thinks for Parkinson's, and that only made things worse.

"She would get sick and upchuck clear across the room. We tried that for a couple months."

He was getting desperate. He asked Sonny to find another doctor, and eventually, they met with Dr. Sakkubai Naidu, the director of Neurogenetics at the Kennedy Kreiger Institute in Baltimore, a short walk from Hopkins. Dr. Naidu worked as a research scientist in neurogenetics. She was also a Professor of Neurology and Pediatrics at the Johns Hopkins University School of Medicine, and like Dr. Johnson, she was well-trained and well-traveled.

In 1962, she graduated from the Madras Medical College in India. She worked at Albert Einstein College of Medicine in the Bronx and three other hospitals before coming to Hopkins in 1984 as a Joseph P. Kennedy, Jr. Foundation Scholar.

She took a keen interest in Patsy's case, and Patsy liked her quite a bit.

Mike says, "Dr. Nadiu asked Sonny if he knew anything about his family tree. I believe Sonny was doing a lot of the family tree before this even started. Dr. Nadiu started comparing the stories to what Sonny was saying about his mother, what symptoms and everything, and one day all of us went down to Dr. Nadiu, and she had a chalkboard, and she had the names on there and compared what happened to Patsy's mother.

"Besides Patsy's mother, Dr. Naidu figured that somebody else in the family had that same disease. The doctor talked to Sonny mostly, because I couldn't understand all the medical terms, and Sonny must have read up on a lot of this stuff, because Sonny knew what she was talking about. And I didn't understand it. Even to this day, I don't understand it."

It's all very complicated, but it helps to understand a bit about brain cells. There are two basic types, neurons and glia. Neurons get all the publicity. They're the famous brain cells. We've each got about 100 billion, and each of those 100 billion can have thousands of connections to the others. Neurons receive signals on dendrites, which sort of resemble tree branches connected to the cell body. Each neuron can have many dendrites coming in, but only one axon going out.

Axons can be quite long. The longest reaches from the bottom of our spines to our toes. What we typically call a nerve is actually a bundle of axons, sheathed in their own myelin, and wrapped together in layers of connective tissue.

Glia is derived from the Greek word for "glue." For a long time, scientists thought the glial cells were there solely to support the neurons. Now they think there's a lot more to it and that most likely both the neurons and glial cells are vital for proper brain communication.

Dr. Tamargo reported "prominent degeneration of the white matter with gliosis and fragmented axons." Gliosis refers to scarring in the central nervous system caused by brain trauma. Too much scarring leads to permanent damage.

So, Patsy had damaged myelin, damaged axons, and extensive scarring, adding up to a brain that could no longer send, receive, and process information in a way that would enable normal life.

Dr. Nadiu identified Patsy's disease as one of the leukodystrophies, namely Hereditary Diffuse Leukoencephalopathy with Spheroids.

Eventually, the people who decide these things, changed the name to "Adult-onset leukoencephalopathy with axonal spheroids and pigmented glia (ALSP)."

In 2016, the *European Journal of Neurology*, the official journal of the European Academy of Neurology, published an extensive study of the disease based on 90 families and 120 cases.

According to the study, the disease "causes dementia, psychiatric symptoms, parkinsonism, seizures and other neurological symptoms and typically begins when patients are in their 40s and 50s."

They define psychiatric symptoms as "anxiety, depression, apathy, indifference, abulia, irritability, disinhibition, and distraction."

Neurologists use the term abulia to describe an absence of initiative, a lack of will.

Under motor dysfunction, the report talks of "parkinsonian symptoms, gait disturbances, spasticity," and difficulty finding words or even speaking. They also mention dizziness, fatigue, and epilepsy and point out that many patients, particularly younger women, and especially early on, are misdiagnosed with multiple sclerosis.

All of this sounds very familiar.

Dr. Nadiu was able to label the disease with confidence, but despite all the evidence indicating ALSP, she could not point to a specific gene to prove her diagnosis.

The gene for ALSP wasn't discovered until 2012. The National Library of Medicine maintains a website called the Genetic Home Reference, which states that "leukoencephalopathy with neuroaxonal spheroids and pigmented glia" is "caused by mutations in the *CSF1R* gene." *CSF1R* is short for colony stimulating factor 1 receptor, and according to the NIH website, "More than a dozen mutations in the *CSF1R* gene have been found in people with adult-onset leukoencephalopathy with axonal spheroids and pigmented glia (ALSP)."

Which brings us briefly to the amazing and complicated topic of genes and chromosomes and deoxyribonucleic acid, which we all know as DNA. DNA is actually an amazingly complex molecule shaped like a very long twisted ladder and stuffed into the nucleus of every cell in every one of us and every other living thing.

The instructions for building each form of life and each member of each form are written in this molecule. Every living thing, from bacteria, algae, fungus, ants, Neanderthals, and elephants to humans develops from instructions written in the DNA. In humans, those instructions are passed down from parents, who got them from their parents, who got them from their parents, in these little packages called chromosomes.

We have 23 pairs of chromosomes. We get one of each chromosome from each parent for a total of 46 chromosomes. Each chromosome contains a distinct section of our total DNA, and within these sections our 20 to 25 thousand genes are defined. If you think of DNA as a language, each chromosome contains a library of books written in that language, and each gene is one of those books.

The *CSF1R* gene resides on the fifth chromosome. Helen got one of these chromosomes from Harry and one from Annie. Most likely, one of them contained the mutations that caused the disease.

It's extremely complex how a cell reads and executes the instructions in its genes, but regardless of the amazing biochemical mechanics, each cell does get its instructions from the DNA in its nucleus and executes them. If something is wrong with the instructions, or if something is wrong in the execution of the instructions, terrible things can happen.

There's a lot more to be said about all this, questions about how Helen got the gene to begin with. Was it passed down through the family? If so, then how and by whom? What was it that Dr. Nadiu saw in the family history? (We have been unable to contact Dr. Nadiu.)

But we're not going to answer these questions. That would be another book. However, we can at least speculate about another interesting question. Why did the disease strike Helen in her thirties and

Patsy in her fifties? They both displayed most of the symptoms typically associated with the disease, but it hit Helen much earlier.

According to the *European Journal of Neurology* report, out of 120 cases studied, the mean age of onset in women was 40. The mean from onset to incapacitation was 3.9 years, and from onset to death was 6.8. If Helen's was an average case, although her onset was early, the other numbers match up well with what we know about her life and the progress of the disease and would indicate that Helen's disease probably started around 1946 when she was 33.

By email, I asked Dr. David Bernard of the National Human Genome Research Institute (NHGRI) in Bethesda what factors might cause the differences in time of onset between Helen and her daughter. Dr. Bernard, who worked on the project that successfully sequenced the human genome, wrote at length about the disease and the *CSFR1* gene and the proteins involved in successful execution of the gene's instructions (called gene expression), as well as the various ways things might have gone wrong.

But when it came to differences in the age of onset, he also said that factors other than pure genetics were most likely involved.

He wrote, "Environmental factors such as stress, other health conditions, smoking, alcohol consumption, diet or exercise could exacerbate, or compensate for, the mutation and change the age of onset of the disease. Just because you have a genetic variation that increases the likelihood of a heart attack doesn't mean you will have a heart attack."

At Springfield, they reported that the visitors from Helen's family blamed Whitey for what happened to Helen. Sid's cousin Shirley blames Whitey, too. So did Shirley's mother. So did her aunt Thelma, her grandmother Devona, and her great aunts, Nan and Esther.

One of Sid's brothers recently said, "Our father made our mother crazy."

There could be a case for that. Maybe her early onset was triggered by her situation, by the loneliness, anxiety, resentment, stress.

Maybe it was Whitey who woke up the monster lurking in Helen's genes.

And maybe it struck Patsy at a later age because Patsy was a happy person with a husband who was her best friend. She had horses and interests and freedom. She had no children and could go wherever she wanted. She had a beautiful home facing a wall of trees climbing a mountain. She had a job she was good at and liked.

Then she got breast cancer. And got treated for it. Did the disease weaken something? Did the treatment? Was the cancer Patsy's Whitey?

We'll never know. But we do know this. Dr. Nadiu said the disease was progressive and incurable. She said Patsy would become an invalid. She would last for some time in a state of complete dependence. And then she would die. Nothing could save her.

She was going to suffer. They were all going to suffer. It was just a matter of time and degree. So, they went home. And they suffered for a long time and to a great degree.

A CHALLENGE OF A LIFETIME

One time I took Patsy back to the bathroom.
I would take her out of the wheelchair and set her on the
commode, and I turned around to the sink to get a
washcloth, and I don't know what she was trying to do,
but she fell off the commode. And when she did,
she reached over and grabbed one of the drawers to the
vanity. And she set there for 45 minutes banging that
drawer. Bang. Bang. Bang. Never left up. And I set down
with her on the floor, and I cried like a baby and tried to
talk to her, but she never left up. Bang. Bang. Bang.

MIKE MCKEE, 2019

I'd say close to a year that we fed her.
We'd have to get her mind on something else probably
about the last two or three months. We'd get the food up
and she'd open her mouth. She knew what was going on
around her, but she couldn't respond.

MIKE MCKEE

Patsy almost never cried. It's possible she didn't even cry when she was born. But that night after falling off the toilet she cried a little.

"I figure she was mad at her situation," Mike says. "And she could do nothing about it. That night she kinda cried, but not what I call cry. She had tears, but Patsy never expressed herself like that. She never complained or talked about her problems. Even when she got breast cancer. I tried to console her, but she didn't want to hear nothing about it. She was going to face it herself and that was it."

At one point, after talking with a friend whose wife also had breast cancer, Mike thought Patsy's chances would be better if she had a mastectomy instead of a lumpectomy. He sat her at the table and made his case. He told her he thought the odds were better for long-term survival if she had the mastectomy.

He talked a long time, but Patsy just sat there like he hadn't said a word. She didn't even look at him. He gave up.

"I can give you a good example of Patsy," Mike says. "I took her fishing, and she put a worm on the hook, and I showed her how to cast, and she took the rod back and hooked me right in the ear. She never asked how I was. Nothing. I mean, nothing.

"I had to go clear back to Clear Spring with a nightcrawler on a hook in my ear, and Uncle Homer had to cut the hook out. And she sat there in the car, while I drove back, like everything was normal. It didn't do no good to get mad at her.

"All the time I ever knew her, she never sobbed. She cried a little bit when her daddy died. I remember it must have been 10 or 11 at night they called her and told her that her daddy passed, and she cried some, but that was it."

Mike brought in a wheelchair. He put in a shower downstairs.

"I put a stool where I could set her to shower and everything. First of all, she was upstairs and had to go up and down the steps, and we had a bathtub upstairs, and she could get in and out of the bathtub. It got to the point where she couldn't get in the tub, and I'd set her in the tub, but then she couldn't get up and down the steps.

"I took the bed and put the bed in the living room, and she just sat and watched TV the last year."

She sat in a blue recliner beside a wall of windows facing out onto the pretty grass and trees behind their house. She could look straight ahead and see a big TV mounted on the wall. She could look to her left and see Mike ride by on the mower during hot summer days, and he could look in and see her in her blue chair.

She stopped talking.

"About a year and a half, she wasn't talking," Mike says. "You could see it coming gradually. Like if I come home from work, I'd talk to her, ask her who all was there in the day, and she would tell me and stuff, but don't get me wrong, the words was slow coming. She had to sit down and kind of think about it."

She spoke clearly when she spoke. She didn't sound like a mute trying to vocalize, the way Dr. Sonnenfeldt described Helen. But each day she spoke less, until one day, Mike realized Patsy didn't talk anymore. He would never hear her voice again and couldn't recall her last words.

She had reached a point similar to Helen's when they moved her to Cottage 5 for custodial care. Or maybe not quite. Like Helen, she couldn't walk, or talk, but she could still think with some clarity. She could control her eyes. And eventually, when everything else was gone, that's how she told Mike what she needed.

He says, "Here's the craziest thing, and I thank God for it. Don't ask me how that I knew, but I could look at her and knew whether she wanted a drink of water, whether she wanted something to eat, whether she wanted the TV changed. I could walk in, and I could ask her, 'What do you want to watch?' Say *The Golden Girls* was on. I don't know how, but I could look at her, and I knowed she wanted to watch something else. And I could put something else on the TV, and I turn around, and the expression in her eyes told me that's what she wanted to watch.

"One time when I mowed, I went by the window, and I had her in that blue chair in there, and she looked at me, and I knowed she wanted a glass of water and come in and give her a glass of water, and that's what she wanted.

"I have no idea how I knew. That was a God sent thing to me and Patsy that I always knew what she wanted. I could look at her and know."

Patsy needed constant attention. Mike worked from four to midnight, so he put together a team. A member of the team was always there. It was Mike and this team who provided the custodial care Helen got in Cottage 5 at Springfield. Only at Springfield, Helen was one of many cared for by very few. Patsy was one cared for by many. And they all knew her and loved her.

Mike says, "I made sure she stayed home. I thought I could really take care of her. She was never alone and never wanted. If she needed a change, she never had to worry about that. If she was hungry or thirsty, she was always taken care of.

"The combination of people that was there, I think, made Patsy live a lot longer than she would have. If she wet herself, they changed her diaper."

Jane Fisher told me, "Mike would have the whole group up to visit with Pat. Mike is a pretty good cook, and he would have quite a spread for us. And we would sit around the table, and of course, Pat would be all happy to see us. And Mike would entertain us with stories about the prison. He had us laughing, and Pat was laughing.

"I remember the last time I saw her. I knew Mike had caregivers staying with her when he was at work. I think I was out shopping, and just on the spur of the moment, I said, 'I'm gonna go up and see Pat.'

"Mike was already gone, but the caregiver was there, and I'd never met this lady, but she was very nice. Pat was sitting in the recliner in the living room. The caregiver and I were talking, but I was also talking to Pat, and I would say, 'Remember Bill? Remember Tom?'

"These were the guys she used to carry on with in our department, and she'd go 'yeah,' and she'd even mention 'John,' and I said 'yeah, John.' She remembered the names, but she didn't really communicate a lot with me. I would remind her of stories, and she'd laugh, and that was probably the last time I saw her.'"

After that conversation, Jane told me to call anytime. I told her I would. She was so nice, and she really liked talking about Patsy, even though it made her cry. And I had so many more questions, but one day, I got a text from Sid.

"Jack, Jane Fisher passed away today."

I don't think she was sick when we spoke. If she was, maybe she didn't know it. She died much more quickly than Patsy did. Whenever I think of her, I think of Vince Vance and the Valiants singing about love and Christmas over a small radio in Patsy's cubicle.

One day, Sid and I visited Mike. We sat at the table in his dining room. Mike showed us pictures. I could see Sid absorbing it all with a sort of amazed emotion, whispering every now and then, "It's so tragic," or just, "Wow."

There's a great picture of Mike with a full head of dark hair, smiling and looking at the camera. Then comes Charlie right beside him. Then comes Dee, another horse. And then Patsy. Patsy's hair is curly and brown. She's wearing glasses and smiling with an arm around Dee. Mike has his arm around Charlie. It's a happy family.

There's a small photo album Mike brought out for us. In one picture, Patsy's in the blue chair. Her sisters are on either side of her, Beverly on her left, Betty on her right. They're each holding one of Patsy's hands and smiling at the camera. Patsy's hair is short and straight. It's dark. She's wearing glasses and sitting between her sisters. Maybe she's trying to smile, but she can't anymore.

There's one picture where Beverly holds a spoon to Patsy's mouth. And there's one that's just Patsy. Someone took off her glasses. She's alone on the blue chair, facing someone's camera. Her skin is some off color. Her eyes are haunting. There's no hint of a smile. It's this picture that reminds me of the picture of Kate Sterling, who would have been Patsy's great grandmother.

Sid looks at it and shakes his head, and then, just above a whisper, he says, "Mike, she's really sick here. She's really sick."

Sid's voice is soft, amazed, and very sad. There's a date on the back of the picture. It's December of 2004. It's a Christmas gathering.

And Sid whispers, "She's dying."

But not yet.

Mike brought in an electric bed that he could raise or lower so Patsy could sit up and watch TV. Her life was the electric bed, the blue chair, and the television.

Mike says, "Patsy loved *The Golden Girls* and *I Love Lucy*. And here's what was really crazy. She would set and laugh. But that's the only thing she could laugh at. *I Love Lucy* and *The Golden Girls*. She knew what was going on with the TV.

"I'd say close to a year that we fed her. We'd have to get her mind on something else, probably about the last two or three months. We'd get the food up, and she'd open her mouth. She knew what was going on around her, but she couldn't respond.

"That was another crazy thing. She never ate breakfast when she was working and stuff. But then I started fixing breakfast. I'd fix her pancakes with blueberries and pecans. And she'd eat three or four every morning when she was sick. Before, she'd never eat a thing.

"Either I'd feed her, or the girls who were there. We'd have to get her mind on other things. I guess sidetracked is what I want to say. She'd open her mouth and we'd be able to feed her. The last couple months were the roughest. You could really see her go downhill."

One day she stopped eating. Shortly afterward, she went into a home hospice program. A nurse would come to the house and check on her. The hospice people brought in monitors. Mike could watch the beat of her heart on a little screen.

Two weeks after she stopped eating, on March 1, 2006, things started shutting down. It was a Wednesday afternoon.

There was a nurse there all the time now, and Patsy must have been in some kind of pain, but Mike doesn't really remember. He just knows she was on morphine at the end for about a week.

"The hospice nurses controlled the morphine. They kept her what's called 'comfortable.'"

That Wednesday, the hospice nurse told Mike it would happen soon. Sonny came over with Lois. Beverly came and Aunt Leila.

Patsy was 56. Her heart rate went up and down on the monitor. Her brain sent a few final messages out into the void, where they died in a wasteland of frayed axons and ruined myelin. Nothing answered. The hospice nurse called them in.

It wasn't quick. Mike says, "I kept waiting and waiting, and Sonny told me to go up and catch a nap, and they would keep watch."

Mike went upstairs and tried to sleep. He was exhausted, but it wasn't long till Sonny came and got him.

He says, "I come down, and I was there no more than five minutes."

The beats on the monitor slowed down. There were long pauses between them.

"You could watch her breathing. And her heart rate just kept dropping and dropping."

Then it went still. It was three hours after midnight.

By law, the nurse could not declare her dead. They called, and the coroner came, and then Patsy was dead.

Mike called the funeral home. And they came. They made Mike leave the room as they prepared to carry her out.

"They didn't want me to watch that. I went back up in the room, and well, I bawled my guts out."

Mike cried more in those few minutes than Patsy had in 56 years.

He says, "We never took a vacation."

He says, "She lived four and a half years after Dr. Johnson told us a year and half."

He says she was in there till the end. "She would set there and laugh at the TV."

They buried her on Friday the third, two days after she died. The family asked that instead of flowers, well-wishers donate to the Hospice of Washington County. People sent flowers anyway. There's an envelope filled with flower cards, most addressed to Patsy's second parents, Beverly and Raymond Stenger on Walnut Point West in Hagerstown.

Mike gave me everything he has. All the records. All the cards. All the facts he could gather. There's a big envelope filled with things, remnants of unpleasant tasks, bad memories, and brutal responsibilities, a record of a sad day in a sad time when sad people did their small bit. There's a tabulation of expenses for the McKee luncheon on March 6, 2006.

A half pan of mac and cheese for $50, miscellaneous groceries, soda and creamer and rolls, $119.05 total, all neatly tabulated down to the nickel on a piece of paper by someone with a broken heart and neat handwriting 15 years ago.

There's a list of pall bearers. There's a list of names and the things people will bring and do. Sandy Tedrick with banana bread. Bill Tedrick with chicken. Louise Stottlemeyer with cake and slaw, lots of volunteers to help with the kitchen. A lot of fruit salad, too, and cake and brownies, and everyone will eat, and everyone will clean up, and everyone will hate it.

There's information about shampoo troughs ($25) and hospital beds, about advance directives and disposal tips for home health care, what to do with needles and syringes and soiled bandages.

There's a letter from a lawyer reminding the McKees that he sent the proposed drafts of their last wills and testaments. He wants to know if the documents are acceptable. They're still there in their long, thick, narrow envelopes, glued tightly shut. Never opened. As they'll stay.

Beverly loved her young sister. She loved her as a sister. She loved her as a daughter. She watched over her and raised her and suffered terribly through her long illness, much like Nan suffering through Helen's.

And then she handled her loss with grace and dignity. She wrote letters to everyone who helped them. She wrote the pall bearers. She wrote the women who spent their days keeping Patsy company while Mike worked. The letters were deeply thoughtful.

Dear Blanche,

On behalf of Mike and all of us in the McKee and Starliper families, we want to do our best to thank you for the care that you lovingly provided to Patsy during the long years of her illness. We will never forget your reliable, skillful, and compassionate attention. You always brought us a smile. We don't know what we would have done without you.

We know how hard it was to do all you did, both physically and emotionally. Only those of us who participated in this most difficult of times at Patsy's side can appreciate your contribution. It was a challenge of a lifetime. Your indomitable spirit and smile were always welcome and a part of the support and morale that kept Patsy and us going. You have meant more to us than we can fairly describe.

We know that Patsy would want to thank you many times over for your gentleness and friendship as well as for your help in these trying years. God bless you.

Love,

Beverly Stenger

In *The Seven Starlipers of Clear Spring*, Sonny wrote, "She was the kindest, sweetest, happiest, most generous, loving, and prettiest of God's creations and the shining light in our eyes."

He wrote, "Nothing has ever shaken and shocked and stole so much from us as did her passing. It is impossible to describe Mike's love and unfailing dedication to Patsy's comfort during the period of her illness of roughly 5 years of bitterly painful and heart wrenching slow cold deterioration. He did all any spouse could do and more, if that is possible. And he did it while every day maintaining the cheerfulness with Patsy that was so steadfast it was hard to believe...

"Even Dr. Nadiu volunteered to me more than once, shaking her head, that she was amazed by Mike's dedication and his almost unprecedented success in keeping Patsy at home through the entire ordeal.

"We will always keep in our hearts her smile, boundless generosity, almost constant joking, and her universe of happiness entirely within her own home and family."

By the time he died, twelve years later, it's likely Sonny had never gotten over Patsy's death.

HELEN AND PATSY

Patsy died at 56. Helen died over half a century earlier at 39. They died in the same state in separate counties in separate centuries. Their time together was short. They shared a single moment of great drama that no one witnessed, a silent birth in the dark.

When Patsy died, it had been over five years since she began dragging her foot and 55 since her mother began dragging hers. They never held a conversation. They loved each other, but they never knew each other.

Helen was the seventh child in her family. Patsy was the seventh in hers. They were both unplanned and unexpected. They began their lives as the babies of their families, helpless and dependent. They ended their lives the same way.

At his table the day Sid and I looked at pictures of Patsy sitting in her blue chair, I asked Mike how he felt when it finally ended.

He said, "Lost."

And then, after a second, "I'm still lost. Everybody says about finding another woman, but I had the woman I loved. That's the bottom line. Me and Patsy, we had a special love and a special marriage. I think about it all the time. I mean look here."

He pointed around the house. There was a guitar he'd never learned to play sitting untuned on a stand. The carpets were clean, and everything seemed in place.

"When Patsy died that's the way it was right here. Nothing's changed."

But really, everything's changed. It just hasn't moved.

Sonny, Beverly, Betty, Bob, Sid, and Dave lost their mother to a disease so rare it barely exists. It had no name, and no one knows when and how it came into existence. They lost their sister to the same thing.

One day at Betty's kitchen table, Sid said, "By watching our sister die, we got to watch our mother die."

At first, no one really cared that much about how their mother died. But then Sonny did and then Sid, and it turns out that really, secretly, they all cared, they were all deeply affected by it, even though they never spoke about it.

Helen wasn't there to raise them, but she did her best to give them a good start. They may not remember her, but she lives on in every one of them, curled up in the nucleus of the 30 trillion cells that make up their bodies.

If Patsy hadn't been born, the disease might have died at Cottage 5 in Springfield's Epileptic Colony. Patsy didn't have any children, so maybe they buried it when they buried her, at least the version carried in the genes of this family.

Helen died with a burning fever, pneumonia, and bed sores, surrounded by strangers in a place filled with the old and sick and mostly forgotten. Patsy died in the electric bed in her living room, surrounded by people who loved her. She went quietly. There was morphine. There were monitors and digital readouts and the faint beeps of modern machines.

There was no last smile. And she did not speak.

After Patsy's funeral, Mike went home. He was 57. He had no kids, no horses, no dogs that pointed with their tails. The blue chair was empty. The TV was dark.

He went back to the prison. Another five and a half years. Another 2,000 days. Coming home at sunrise to a home where no one made red velvet cakes anymore.

Then he retired. Ten years after Patsy's funeral, Sid invited Mike to a gathering in honor of Patsy's mother. And during that gathering in Sid's yard, Mike pulled aside a piece of cloth that covered a painting, and there she was.

Today the painting hangs on the wall beside a picture in black and white of young Patsy and her young brother Dave, with big smiles and big front teeth, holding a cat named Fluffy between them. The painting's right beside the blue chair where she spent the last year of her life. The chair faces the wall and the big dark silent TV that hasn't played *The Golden Girls* since 2006.

"IT'S OKAY"

Patient was able to talk.

SPRINGFIELD HOSPITAL, OCTOBER 5, 1952

"It's okay. It's okay."

HELEN STARLIPER, JANUARY 26, 2020

As January neared its end in 2020, they finally came out to the canal and tore down Helen's home. Sid sent me an email from the spot.

"It's a sad, sad day for me."

It was a Sunday afternoon. I was at the museum in Sykesville, and he was out where the house wasn't anymore, looking at their work. They were probably just a crew of guys with noisy machines and a job to do. It was a demolition job, not an archeological expedition. Their mission was to remove the last evidence of a forgotten past to make the present more safe and attractive.

They didn't know about Bob Small going off to war from that house in 1918, or Ann Reid walking out one morning to meet her destiny in the form of a ram. They didn't know about Harry Small's head hitting the ground, or the terrible thing that happened to the baby of the family.

A family lived in that rubble. Only one family. Ever. Seven children were born there. One died in an institution.

They tore it down and hauled it away. Sid walked around what wasn't there anymore and cried.

And then one of those strange things happened, like Bob Evans.

A few days later, sitting around a table with me and his ex-wife, Karen, in the quiet of the Gate House Museum, Sid told us about it. He was quite emotional as he talked and had to stop now and then to compose himself, much like Jane Fisher talking about Patsy. He looked off past me into the distance.

"On that Sunday morning," he says, "I drove up to mom's place on the river, because I had been told that the house was torn down, and I wanted to go see it. So, I went up there and I parked my car in front of what used to be the old barn.

"And I could tell already that the house was gone. So, I walked back down to the front of the house, and they had put up a safety fence preventing you from driving in there, a little orange fence, and I walked around that safety fence.

"I picked up my phone, because I wanted to take a picture, but I was too close, so I walked across the road to the other side and took a picture from there. And then I went back and around the fence and walked up to the foundation, and they had filled the cellar in with fresh dirt, and they had covered it with a fabric mulch-type material.

"So, that's when...it's kind of hard for me to talk about...that's when I said to myself, 'Mom's house is gone. It's gone.'

"So, I walked across the parlor, and the ground was real soft, and I had trouble walking, because my feet were sticking in the mud. And...and...so I got across the parlor. And I stepped over to the kitchen. And I'm crying. I'm crying. And I stepped over into the kitchen, and out of nowhere, I hear the words.

"'It's okay. It's okay.'

"I didn't know what was happening. I still don't know what was happening, other than, I didn't really hear the words. The words came into my head. 'It's okay. It's okay.' And they did a nice job.

"I'm not sure if I fabricated the words 'they did a nice job' on my own. I know I did not manufacture or fabricate, 'it's okay.' And I kept hearing that. 'It's okay. It's okay.'

"At that point, I was sort of like in shock. What's going on? How is it okay? I stopped crying. And it is okay. It's okay. They did a nice job. They didn't destroy the foundation. The footprint is there. It's almost like I did it myself.

"So, then the phone rang. It was Beth. And Beth said, 'Dad, are you okay?' And I remember trying to tell her. It's okay. They did a good job. They did a nice job. I tried not to use those words, 'it's okay,' but it kept sticking with me.

"They did a nice job. Beth, they did a nice job. So, we talked and talked. The important part for me…how did that happen? Why did that happen? Who was that? Was it an angel?

"I believe in God. Was it God? Was it Helen? Who said, 'It's okay?'

"And I don't know, and I guess I'll never know, and it doesn't matter, except that those words came into my head. There wasn't a voice. I don't remember a voice. Those words came from somewhere. Where did they come from? 'It's okay.'

"And immediately, it's like turning a light on in a dark room. When I stepped from the parlor into the kitchen, and it's not really much of a step, because it's not much of a difference in elevation, everything changed. I don't know how to explain it.

"And I remember, Karen said, 'You shouldn't have been over there alone.' But I wasn't alone. After I stepped into the kitchen, everything was fine. I was fine. And I couldn't wait to go down the back to the river and look down at the canal boats. Of course, not the canal boats, but the towpath, and it turned out to be a wonderful day. The house was gone, but it was okay."

At that point, Karen said to me, "I think it was a spiritual experience. Sid has struggled so through this, even as good as it's all been, it's still a struggle, and I just feel like God gave him that ability to let go right there in that moment, and it couldn't have been a more perfect place."

Sid says, "You see, when I went up the steps in 2016, and I looked up at the sky, there wasn't any roof, right? And I'm thinking, I'm in mom's bedroom, and it's a good place to die. That was my words.

"'It's okay,' that was not my words. They were not my words."

A long time ago, when we were just getting started, Sid said, "Maybe someday in some far corner of the world, someone will read this story, and it will help them somehow."

That would be nice, but here's what I think about. Just like men with machines came and erased her house, Helen's life had nearly been erased. No one spoke of her. There were very few pictures of her. She was a forgotten woman with a forgotten grave, no stone, just a plate flat on the ground in an unknown cemetery in a town no one heard of.

But now, her son can walk into Bob Evans in Frederick, or any of the other 470 or so Bob Evans around the country, and he can show everyone in there a book with his mother's picture on it and her story inside. And at night, before he goes to bed, he can pick that book up. He can run his fingers through the pages and read about her. He can look at Helen's face when she was young and happy and had no idea something invisible was working against her. He can look at a picture of Helen and Thelma by a fence with their dresses blowing in the wind way back during the Depression.

He can know that once in her life, there were walks up into the mountains, where Helen, Thelma, and Genevieve, and all their little kids, ate flaming marshmallows and hot dogs on sticks. He can know that, once in her life, there were banjos and fiddles and carnivals and big slides into the river at Row's park, and a handsome guy named Whitey slugging it out with guys named Kid and Powerhouse and Red. And there was square dancing to Joe Mills and his Fiddlers. And Helen danced with Thelma and Genevieve. And they loved her. And Nan loved her. Lots of people loved her. And when she talked, they heard music.

The canal's beautiful now. Thousands go by Helen's backyard every year. They walk and they run. They ride fancy bikes. On sunny summer afternoons, they zip and bounce around the river behind her house with loud machines that stink up the air. They swim and shout and drink beer and party and jump off the towpath into the river.

They have no idea she's up there, high up that cliff in the trees and the rocks and the soft dirt over the kitchen and over those two old stairways that are buried now, side by side in that dirt, like a pair of dinosaurs.

When they took down the house, they cut the sweet shrub to the level of the earth. They didn't get the roots. It's alive. And the big hunk that Sid stole and stuck out the window of his car, it's alive, too. It sprouts its flowers by the arbor in his yard, and another one sprouts its flowers in Betty's yard. And when every member of Helen's family and Sid's and all the rest of us are gone, that shrub will keep growing at the edge of the Potomac by the ghost of a vanished house.

And before he goes to bed each night, Sid can say, "Good night, Mom, I love you." And maybe she hears. And maybe she says, "Thanks, Sidney. I love you, too."

It's nice to think so. And he does. And finally, after all this time and all he's learned about the things that happened to his mother 70 years ago, Sid knows that they happened then and can't be changed and aren't happening now.

Whatever she suffered, she suffered a long time ago.

It's over. She's gone. And it's okay.

"It's okay."

AFTERWORD

Whitey

I think it's important to say a bit more about Whitey, because we left his life sort of unfinished, and there's more to tell.

Obviously, he was a weak father and a terrible husband. No one defends him. His kids don't speak kindly of him. Some are harder on him than others. Some don't forgive him at all.

But he did change after Helen died, not immediately, and not because she died. For one thing, he stopped drinking so much.

"He married this woman, and she had three children of her own. They lived in her house in Hagerstown," Sid says.

The woman was Gladys. Dave, Bob, and Sid would visit. Gladys treated them well.

When he lived with Gladys, Whitey raised a garden. He drove an old car that he painted with a brush. When Sid was 15 or so, they borrowed a plow from a farmer and attached it to the car with a rope and used that car to plow his garden.

"He turned his life around," Sid says. "He was not the ideal father, but he certainly wasn't drinking every night, like he was when he was with our mother. He had a steady job. He worked at that meat market in the west end of Hagerstown.

"We got along really well, and that was kind of hidden away, this thing with mom. We would visit each other, and I'd help him, and he helped me, but we never talked about her.

"Back in the sixties, we worked together in Gaithersburg as carpenters. Daddy had that old pickup that was rusted so bad you could see the asphalt on the road. I should have realized his situation. I wasn't rich, but I had enough. I could have helped him, but I never did. I always felt guilty that I never helped him financially.

"I remember him telling me how much gas his little old lawnmower used. It was just a little tiny tank. I remember him complaining about the lawnmower using so much gas, and the cost of gas, and I thought, 'Sid, you big dummy, you didn't help your daddy.'

"He changed completely, and that's a big question. What brought about that change? Did Gladys change him? I don't know.

"Sonny told me they were in the car together one day, and Daddy said something like, 'I wasn't a very good father. I guess I didn't do very good by you kids,' or something like that, and Sonny agreed with him."

Gladys died, and Whitey married again, and then again. He died in his late seventies of prostate cancer. There's a picture of him with Patsy at her wedding. They both have big smiles. And when he died, and she got the call, that was the first time Mike saw Patsy cry.

Sid went to a car show in Carlisle, Pennsylvania, recently with his brothers Bob and Dave. It's something the four brothers had done for years. Now there are three. Sid told his brothers he's tried to hate his father, but he just can't do it.

Bob told him, "Sid, you just don't have it in you."

"I love my daddy," Sid says.

Peachie

She didn't make it. She had the stage 4 cancer, and after she broke her pelvis, Peachie only lasted a few more weeks. She was smart and talented, with a gigantic laugh, and except for Sid (and me), no one wanted more to have this book completed.

She got to see a proof. She smiled when Sid showed it to her, but she was on strong painkillers and probably didn't understand what she was looking at. Her reading days were over.

Her real name was Mary Ida. Her father, who was gassed during the First World War, gave her the nickname. She was born in Clear Spring in 1928 and buried there on October 17, 2020.

In 1949, Peachie moved to Allentown, Pennsylvania, where she had seven children with her first husband, Tom Morgan, helped found a library, and ran her own bridal shop. After her husband passed away, she married Guy Haines in 1991. Guy was her high school sweetheart, and they met again at a Clear Spring High School reunion.

She made amazing quilts. She won awards at rose shows. She volunteered at the Plumb Grove farmhouse museum in Clear Spring, where she researched long-forgotten heritage roses from the 18th and 19th centuries. Eventually, she planted and raised over 130 of these roses on the grounds at the museum.

At her funeral, they asked Sid to say a few words. There was a big crowd, and Sid was nervous. He asked the minister to stand up there with him.

"I did the best that I could," he says.

One week after the funeral, we published the book. I wish she could have read it.

Acknowledgements

I'm especially grateful to my wife, Andrea, who designed the cover and the interior. She also copy-edited the book twice with annoying precision and did all the work necessary to get the book live on Amazon.com.

I'd like to thank Karen Starliper for her support, her insight, and very helpful editing. I'd like to thank Sid's siblings, Beverly, Betty, Dave, and Bob, for feeding me cake and iced tea and telling me stories, many of them very funny, about their mother, their father, their grandmother, their aunts and uncles and each other.

I'd like to thank Guy Haynie (no relation to Guy Haines), for his tales about working at the hospital in the late forties, Jeff Barnes and the late Jack Egolf, for similar tales about a later time, and Annie Boteler for her great interviews with Dr. Kurt Glaser and other Springfield old-timers.

I'd like to thank Ann Horvath, Adrienne Smith, and Mandy Bernard for their help at the museum while I wrote this book. All smart, funny people.

And finally, I'd like to thank my friend, Jon Herman, for getting us into the buildings over at Springfield, even if they were the wrong buildings.

Sid would like to thank Jonathan, too, as well as Springfield Hospital Superintendent Paula Langmead for kindly walking him around the Springfield grounds that day, and Theresa Ronayne, who drove him all over the campus on one of his first visits, when he was somewhat lost and confused. He's also especially grateful to the women in the old Springfield barn who helped him get Helen's records, especially Michelle Stokes who tracked Helen's records down through 800 rolls of microfilm over the course of many months.

He would like to thank Karen Gray of the Chesapeake and Ohio Canal National Historical Park for teaching him a bit about the old canal (including the fact that "there's nothing romantic about a canal boat"), and David Sorflaten for having him over and discussing his early days growing up at Springfield.

He would also like to thank Bernie Henson for his friendship and his bat, Harriet Clopper, David Wiles, and finally, his cousins, Sally Boswell and Shirley Talhelm with their great memories and steel-trap minds.

And of course, he loves and thanks his brothers and sisters, who lived it all with him.

THE FAMILY

Siblings are listed in birth order by their nicknames. Only family members who figure prominently in this book are included.

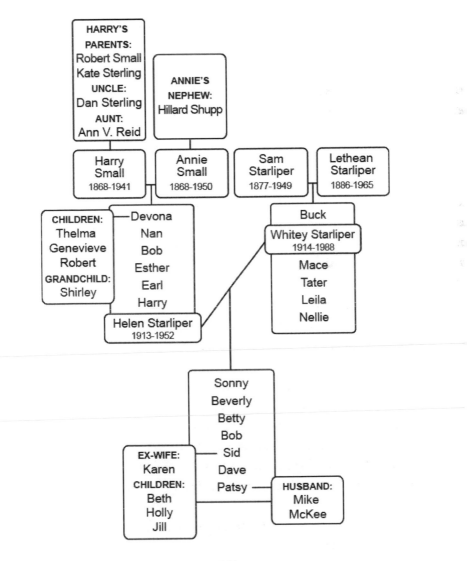

AUTHOR'S NOTES

To put this story together, I relied on interviews, old newspapers and articles, the archives at the Gate House Museum, Helen's medical records, Patsy's medical and personal records, a few contemporary magazines and books, various Starliper family genealogies, the writings of Charles "Sonny" Starliper, and of course, the Internet.

Interviews

I did many interviews with Sid. You might say our relationship during the past two and a half years has been one long interview. I also interviewed Sid's ex-wife, Karen Starliper, on several occasions, always with Sid present.

I never met Sonny, who passed away not long after we got started, but I did interview Sid's brothers Bob and Dave and his sisters Beverly and Betty, all of whom have different perspectives on things. We did these interviews as a group in sessions at Betty's house.

I interviewed Peachie Haines and her husband Guy, Harriet Clopper Haines (Harriet and Peachie are married to brothers), and David Wiles, of the Clear Spring Historical Association, in an 1829 log home called Brown's Meeting House in Clear Spring.

I also interviewed Peachie twice by phone. I interviewed Jane Fisher by phone from my father's house in Philadelphia. In the kitchen at the Gate House, I interviewed Guy Haynie, not to be confused with Guy Haines (Peachie's husband), about his work at Springfield during the late forties. Very few people who worked there then are alive now.

I interviewed Shirley Talhelm by phone. She has an amazing memory and a talent for pulling together beautiful descriptive passages with just the right details straight out of her head.

I have listened to interviews Sid recorded with David Sorflaten at David's home in Rock Creek, Maryland, and with Dr. David Brewer's daughter and son in Clear Spring.

I interviewed Mike McKee on three occasions.

I interviewed Dr. David Bernard of the National Human Genome Research Institute. Dr. Bernard worked on the Human Genome Project that sequenced the entire human genome between 1990 and 2003.

I also interviewed Alice G. Lee, Ph.D, the LaMoyne Professor of Biology at Washington & Jefferson College, who directed the Biology department at the college for six years, and founded the Biochemistry major and ran it for five years.

Newspaper Articles

I did not spend a lot of time researching old newspapers, mainly because Sid did that for me. He sent me a steady supply of articles from old Hagerstown papers.

Mainly these articles were short bits ("The Two Locks Letter," "The Clear Spring Letter," etc.) about the family (picnics, dances, parties, porkers, weenie roasts). There were also full articles, most of which involved tragedies and had headlines like, "Fall Fatal to Aged Man," which described Harry Small's death.

There are many articles about Whitey's various fights and some about his adventures enforcing the law, which weren't nearly as exciting as his father's adventures.

There are far too many articles about the family to list, so I've just listed those articles that provide information that is not directly related to the story of the Starlipers and not taken from the Hagerstown papers.

Armacost, Elise. "A New Life in a New Land." *Carroll County Times*, June 25, 1986. (This is the story of Eva Salomon.)

Brecher, Ruth, and Edward Brecher. "Patients on Parole." *Saturday Evening Post*, 1955.

Shank, Christopher. "Wings Over Hagerstown: Experiencing the Second World War in Western Maryland." *Maryland Historical Magazine*, 1993.

Sorflaten, David. "Remembering Days of Youth at Springfield." *The Evening Sun*, Feb 12, 1982.

Gate House Museum Archives

The Gate House Museum Archives surely sound more impressive than they are, but we do have a huge collection of pictures taken at Springfield over the years, the great majority of which are only in digital form. We also have quite a few documents, including several oral histories by Annie Boteler with men and women who worked at Springfield in some capacity.

Most useful was William Trombley's 1953 analysis of the *Baltimore Sun's* handling of the so-called "Maryland's Shame" series. The original articles were meant to shock. Trombley's article, analyzing the original articles, was actually more well-written, more interesting, and immensely more helpful and informative than the "Maryland's Shame" articles themselves.

Another helpful document was our copy of the report the state put together following their own investigation of the various allegations made in these articles.

The script for William Shipley's talk to a local Rotary Club in 1953 was also very helpful. It provided a detailed, dollar-by-dollar stream of facts down to the annual milk output of various cows (or so it seemed).

Before Dr. Ellis Margolin left the institution in the seventies, he wrote a very helpful farewell letter describing his days at Springfield, obviously with no idea that someday he would be in a book.

Also enjoyable, and very useful, were the writings of David Sorflaten. He published articles in the *Baltimore Sun* and *Carroll County Times*, but the best information is in a long letter he wrote to me describing his days growing up at Springfield, where he lived for the first 18 years of his life.

The archives include a few aborted attempts at a history of the hospital (mostly plagiarized from each other). They include many annual reports by various superintendents, as well as textbooks for nurses, new employee instruction manuals, a detailed explanation of how to process a patient into the institution, detailed nursing instruction manuals and coursework, and also how to take a history from a relative.

I found a notebook with the handwritten notes of a new nurse from 1950, detailing various procedures, including how to handle a dead body immediately after expiration. I decided not to include this information, which I found very interesting, mainly because it was upsetting and seemed like something the book could do without.

And finally, I learned a great deal from the writings of Henrietta DeWitt, who was an influential social worker at Springfield, with great insight into the mentally ill and the difficulties faced by their families, and also from a long document by Mr. Tomlinson, the hospital's assistant supervisor for many years (Mr. Springfield), that provides great insight into how the hospital operated in the days when it was most densely inhabited.

Margolin, E.S., letter to the Superintendent from Pathologist and Director of Laboratories, December 2, 1973, Springfield Hospital Collection, Gate House Museum, Sykesville, Maryland.

Report of the Joint Senate and House Committee of the State Mental Hospitals of Maryland: March, 1949. Springfield Hospital Collection, Gate House Museum, Sykesville, Maryland.

Shipley, William, speech to a local Rotary Club, 1953. (typescript copy). Springfield Hospital Collection, Gate House Museum, Sykesville, Maryland.

Trombley, William. "A Report on the Baltimore Sunpapers' effort to improve conditions in Maryland's mental institutions," (typescript copy written for *Baltimore Sun*, 1953, marked "Tomlinson's copy"). Springfield Hospital Collection, Gate House Museum, Sykesville, Maryland.

Records in Private Collection

I had access to all Helen's records from her arrival at Springfield until her death. The records include the letters of the two doctors who verified Helen's "insanity," and the few brief bits of correspondence between the Starlipers (mainly Lethean) and the hospital.

Mike McKee gave me a much larger collection of medical and personal records for Patsy. Mike and the records don't always agree, but that's because this happened a long time ago, a lot happened, and no one could possibly remember it all in the right order all these years later, especially considering the complexity of the material.

Books

Here's a list of some of the books I read that somehow contributed to my understanding. A couple are actually old college textbooks that I got from Amazon.

The scientific information in these textbooks is almost incomprehensibly amazing, as is everything I learned about human biology while writing this book.

Bauby, Jean-Dominique. *The Diving Bell and the Butterfly.* Vintage International, 1997.

Bryson, Bill. *One Summer: America, 1927.* Anchor Books, 2014.

Bauman, William. *Samuel Sterling Family History.* C&O Canal Association, 2015.

Beam, Alex. *Gracefully Insane.* Public Affairs, 2001.

Bear, Mark F., Barry W. Connors, and Michael A Paradiso. *Neuroscience: Exploring the Brain.* 2nd ed. Lippincott Williams & Wilkins, 2001.

Becker, Wayne M., Lewis J. Kleinsmith, Jeff Hardin, and Gregory Paul Bertoni. *The World of the Cell.* 7th ed. Benjamin Cummings, 2008.

Best, Amy, ed. *How It Works: Book of the Brain.* Future Publishing Unlimited, 2009.

Cahalan, Susannah. *Brain on Fire: My Month of Madness.* Simon & Shuster Paperbacks, 2012.

Clark, Ella E., and Thomas F. Hahn, eds. *Life on the Chesapeake & Ohio Canal, 1859.* American Canal and Transportation Center, 1977.

Dawkins, Richard. *The Selfish Gene.* Oxford University Press, 1976.

Greenberg, Linda F. *Sykesville Past & Present: A Walking Tour.* Brinkmann Publishing, 2012.

Hager, Thomas. *The Demon Under the Microscope.* Three Rivers Press, 2006.

Hahn, Thomas F. *Chesapeake and Ohio Canal Old Picture Album.* American Canal and Transportation Center, 1979.

Hall, Bill. *Images of America: Sykesville.* Arcadia Publishing, 2001.

Kean, Sam. *The Violinist's Thumb.* Little, Brown and Company, 2013.

Kolata, Gina. *Mercies in Disguise.* St. Martin's Press, 2017.

Kytle, Elizabeth. *Home on the Canal.* The Johns Hopkins University Press, 1983.

Lipska, Barbara. *The Neuroscientist Who Lost Her Mind.* Houghton Mifflin Harcourt, 2018.

Marsh, Katharine, ed. *The Great Depression.* Future Publishing Unlimited, 2009.

Murray, T. Jock. *Multiple Sclerosis: The History of a Disease.* Demos Medical Publishing. 2004.

Roberts, Randy. *Joe Louis: Hard Times Man.* Yale University Press, 2010.

Rutherford, Adam, *A Brief History of Everyone Who Ever Lived: The Human Story Retold Through Our Genes.* The Experiment, LLC, 2017.

Time-Life Books, ed. *The Jazz Age: The 20s (Our American Century).* Time-Life Books, 2000.

Unrau, Harlan D. *Historic Resource Study: Chesapeake & Ohio Canal.* National Park Service, 2007.

Walker, William. *Betrayal at Little Gibraltar.* Scribner, 2017.

Whitaker, Robert. *Mad in America.* Basic Books, 2009.

Zimmer, Carl. *She Has Her Mother's Laugh.* Dutton, 2019.

Special Issue Magazines

The Roaring '20s: Flappers, Bootleggers, Gangsters, Suffragists. Single issue magazine, The New York Times, January 1, 2020.

The Roaring '20s: The Decade that Changed America. Single issue magazine, Time-Life, January 6, 2017.

Your Genes: a User's Guide. Special issue magazine, *National Geographic,* January 1, 2019.

Internet

Most of my medical and scientific research, and much of my historical research, took place on the Internet. Below are some particularly useful websites, but it would be impossible to list all the sites I visited over the past three years, as every time I had a question, I went straight to the web.

Codjia, P., X. Ayrignac, and F. Mochei, et. al. "Adult-Onset Leukoencephalopathy with Axonal Spheroids and Pigmented Glia: An MRI Study of 16 French Cases." *American Journal of Neuroradiology.* https://doi.org/10.3174/ajnr.A5744.

"*CSF1R* Gene (Protein Coding)." *GeneCards: The Human Gene Database.* Weizmann Institute of Science. https://www.genecards.org /cgi-bin/carddisp.pl?gene=CSF1R.

Foulds, N., R. Pengelly, and S. Hammans, et al. "Adult-Onset Leukoencephalopathy with Axonal Spheroids and Pigmented Glia Caused by a Novel R782G Mutation in *CSF1R.*" *Scientific Reports,* 5, no. 10042, (2015). https://doi.org/10.1038/srep10042.

"Genetics." *MedlinePlus.* National Institutes of Health: U.S. National Library of Medicine. https://medlineplus.gov/genetics/.

"Hereditary Diffuse Leukoencephalopathy with Spheroids." *Genetic and Rare Diseases Information Center*. National Institutes of Health: National Center for Advancing Translational Sciences. https://rarediseases.info.nih.gov/diseases/10981 /hereditary-diffuse-leukoencephalopathy-with-spheroids.

Kang, Seongsu, Da Mi Kim, In Ho Lee, and Chang June Song. "Adult-onset Leukoencephalopathy with Axonal Spheroids and Pigmented Glia: A Case Report." *Radiology Case Reports*, 14, no. 4, (April 2019): 514-517. https://doi.org/10.1016 /j.radcr.2019.01.021.

Konno, Takuya, Kunihiro Yoshida, and Ikuko Mizuta, et. al. "Diagnostic Criteria for Adult-onset Leukoencephalopathy with Axonal Spheroids and Pigmented Glia Due to *CSF1R* Mutation." *European Journal of Neurology*, 25, no. 1, (2018): 142–147. https://dx.doi.org/10.1111%2Fene.13464.

"Leukodystrophy." National Organization of Rare Diseases (NORD). https://rarediseases.org/rare-diseases/leukodystrophy /#:~:text=Leukodystrophies%20are%20a%20group%20of,myelin %20sheath)%20of%20the%20brain.

"Leukodystrophy Information Page." National Institute of Neurological Disorders and Stroke. https://www.ninds.nih.gov/disorders /all-disorders/leukodystrophy-information-page.

Sundal, C., M. Baker, and V. Karrenbauer, et. al. "Hereditary Diffuse Leukoencephalopathy with Spheroids with Phenotype of Primary Progressive Multiple Sclerosis." *European Journal of Neurology*, 22, no. 2 (2015): 328-333. https://doi.org/10.1111/ene.12572.